COMMUNICATION SKILLS IN NURSING PRACTICE

2ND EDITION

COMMUNICATION SKILLS IN NURSING PRACTICE

EDITED BY
LUCY WEBB

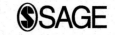

Los Angeles | London | New Delhi
Singapore | Washington DC | Melbourne

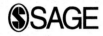

Los Angeles | London | New Delhi
Singapore | Washington DC | Melbourne

SAGE Publications Ltd
1 Oliver's Yard
55 City Road
London EC1Y 1SP

SAGE Publications Inc.
2455 Teller Road
Thousand Oaks, California 91320

SAGE Publications India Pvt Ltd
B 1/I 1 Mohan Cooperative Industrial Area
Mathura Road
New Delhi 110 044

SAGE Publications Asia-Pacific Pte Ltd
3 Church Street
#10-04 Samsung Hub
Singapore 049483

Editor: Alex Clabburn
Assistant editor: Jade Grogan
Production editor: Tanya Szwarnowska
Copyeditor: Nik Prowse
Proofreader: Swales & Willis Ltd, Exeter, Devon
Indexer: Sue Lightfoot
Marketing manager: George Kimble
Cover design: Wendy Scott
Typeset by: C&M Digitals (P) Ltd, Chennai, India
Printed in the UK

This second edition published 2020

First edition published by Oxford University Press 2011

Library of Congress Control Number: 2019943672

British Library Cataloguing in Publication data

A catalogue record for this book is available from
the British Library

ISBN 978-1-5264-8937-1
ISBN 978-1-5264-8936-4 (pbk)

At SAGE we take sustainability seriously. Most of our products are printed in the UK using responsibly sourced
papers and boards. When we print overseas we ensure sustainable papers are used as measured by the PREPS
grading system. We undertake an annual audit to monitor our sustainability.

CONTENTS

PUBLISHER'S ACKNOWLEDGEMENTS

The publishers are grateful to the following academics for their work reviewing both the proposal for the second edition and the revised material.

Peter Ellis, Independent academic, author

Shelly Haslam, Edge Hill University

Michelle Chappell, University of Hull

Karen Cooper, Bournemouth University

Linda Currie, University of York

Gayle Le Moine, Canterbury Christ Church University

PART I
THEORIES OF COMMUNICATION

Preface to Part 1

Communication and interpersonal skills are essential for all nurses, regardless of the area of care. Whether being used for health promotion, building a trusting nurse–patient relationship or delivering a therapeutic intervention, communication and interpersonal skills are the bedrock to delivering patient-centred care, individualised care and patient-led care.

Communication Skills in Nursing Practice has been written for student nurses following pre-registration, nursing associate or apprenticeship programmes. The contributors are all nurses and experienced leaders in their different clinical fields and have years of experience guiding nursing students through education and training. The authors bring up-to-date knowledge and expertise to their topic and demonstrate how theory and practice are linked in the different practice contexts.

There are many books on communication and interpersonal skills available to nursing students. What makes this book different is that it focuses on demonstrating how the theory is applied in practice. Student nurses are taught theory in the academic setting and practice in the clinical setting. This book helps the student bridge the gap between the two. The skills and knowledge addressed here in these chapters reflect the skills expected of all qualifying nurses as detailed in the Nursing and Midwifery Council's *Future Nurse: Standards of Proficiency for Registered Nurses* (NMC, 2018a).

Lucy Webb, Editor

ONE
INTRODUCTION TO COMMUNICATION SKILLS
LUCY WEBB

THE AIMS OF THIS CHAPTER ARE TO:

- Outline the importance of communication skills in nursing
- Explore the underpinning theories and definitions of communication
- Demonstrate theories of communication in the practice setting
- Provide context for the rest of the book

Introduction

Communication is identified as one of the essential skills students must acquire in order to become qualified nurses (NMC, 2018a). This book has been designed to help student nurses understand the underlying reasons why communication skills have become so important in nursing. In all the chapters in this book, you will find examples illustrating how communication is applied in the nursing context. In this way, the book will help you develop your knowledge and skills in order that you feel prepared for practice.

Why is communication important in nursing?

Important skills for the Nursing and Midwifery Council

The Nursing and Midwifery Council (NMC) proficiencies (NMC, 2018a) became effective in 2019 and are split into two key elements: (1) communication and management and (2) nursing procedures. This book specifically addresses the communication and management proficiencies that students will need to demonstrate in order to become registered with the NMC. You will find the full list of communication and management proficiencies in Annex A of the NMC standards document (NMC, 2018a) but, in short, they govern the key skills domains:

1   Underpinning communication skills that enable the practitioner to assess, plan and provide evidence-based practice through:

    a   active listening, non-verbal communication, open and closed questioning
    b   being aware of one's own biases
    c   writing accurate, clear and legible records to share information
    d   analysing and using digital data
    e   recognising the need for translational services.

2   Communication for supporting people of all ages, their families and carers in preventing ill health and in managing their care through:

    a   sharing health information with service users in an understandable way
    b   recognising the need for sensory impairments adjustments and personal communication aids.

3   Use communication to deliver therapeutic interventions and:

    a   be able to use a range of therapeutic techniques where appropriate.

4   Working with professional teams through:

    a   use of effective supervision and teaching/training of staff and students
    b   management of teams through skills in managing change, conflict, negotiation and escalation.

You will find all these competencies addressed throughout this book.

Communication as an aspect of care

We could say that communication skills are linked inextricably to the professional values of nursing. Nurses frequently work the most closely with patients, having a specific position in their role as health professionals to develop and maintain a trusting professional relationship with patients, family members and carers (Fitzpatrick, 2018). Nurses are therefore in the best position to deliver patient-centred care, and to do this compassionately while maintaining the patient's dignity and safety and, of course, effectively. Without effective communication patient care may be negatively affected. Nurses work very closely with the patient but are also heavily involved in the multi-disciplinary team. Therefore, they need to be able to adapt to interact with a wide variety of people. If nurses do not adhere to their professional values, they may put their patients at risk of serious harm. The most crucial point is that behaving and communicating like a professional at all times is vital to becoming a competent nurse. Nurses should never presume things about their patients, and they should use their communication skills to ask relevant questions even about sensitive issues. This enables the nurse to be fully informed about the patient and for them to be able to treat the patient as an individual.

The Royal College of Nursing (RCN) proposes a set of principles that define nursing practice:

1   treat everyone with dignity, humanity and compassion
2   deliver accountable care in collaboration with patients, families and carers
3   manage risk and keep people safe
4   deliver person-centred care, driven by informed choices
5   nurses are at the heart of the communication process involving patients, practitioners and carers
6   nurses have up-to-date knowledge and skills, delivered with intelligence, insight and understanding of patients
7   work with colleagues to provide best possible co-ordinated care
8   nurses lead by example, influencing care that is person-centred.

(RCN, 2018)

These are all skills developed by nurses during their pre-registration education; however, all of them demand good communication skills. It appears that this argument supports the notion that 'nursing', in addition to applied knowledge and caring attitude, is underpinned essentially by communication skills.

The therapeutic effect of good communication is supported by evidence. For instance, Bensing and Verheul (2010) describe communication as 'the silent healer' for its positive effects on how patients experience ill health. Health professionals who can deploy emotional intelligence in their communication develop more effective care relationships and make better care decisions with their patients (Raghubir, 2018). Popa-Velea and Purcărea (2014) list the practical benefits of good communication through facilitating a positive relationship between the practitioner and the patient, allowing the patient to fully explain their needs and enhancing the practitioner's knowledge and understanding of the patient. Street et al. (2009) demonstrate that communication pathways can lead directly to improved health outcomes by delivering health education, motivation and empowerment, and treatment based more closely on the patient's needs.

So, we can see that good communication in the nurse–patient encounter is itself a therapeutic intervention as well as being the vehicle for good care. It is as important as any other care or treatment intervention. In brief, the evidence above suggests that health communication helps patients to:

1   express their physical and emotional needs
2   ask questions and be more involved in their care
3   gain a sense of control over their health and treatment
4   develop trust and confidence in their treatment
5   gain physical health benefits.

The changing nature of healthcare

The changing nature of healthcare itself underlines the importance of good communication. Improved medical treatment over the last century has shifted focus from acute illness to the management of chronic disease. More people are living with survivable chronic illness and therefore need support to be self-caring; for example, managing their own blood sugar levels in diabetes. Because of this shift to chronic care management, quality of life has become as important as survival now that people are living longer with conditions such as cancer, bipolar disorder and physical or learning disability.

This can be referred to as a move from a medical model of healthcare to a biopsychosocial model of healthcare whereby the biological, psychological and social aspects of the patient's wellbeing are taken equally into consideration in a holistic manner to address the patient's quality of life (Ogden, 2012).

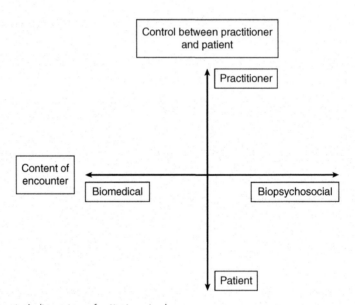

Figure 1.1 Bensing's dimensions of patient-centredness

Overall, there has been a major shift in the relationship between patient and practitioner which has turned the old paternal system of 'doctor knows best' to one of patient-centred care and the 'expert patient'. Bensing's classic work on doctor–patient communication (2000) is summed up in a simple diagram of two dimensions of control and content that dictates the relationship between the patient and the practitioner (see Figure 1.1).

This model maps out the patient–practitioner encounter by who has control of the meeting and how medicalised the communication is. For instance, a visit to the practice nurse may involve the nurse informing the patient that they must take the medication in

order to get better (a practitioner-controlled, medical encounter) or the patient informing the nurse that the side effects are interfering with their work and social life and that
another type needs to be tried (a patient-centred, biopsychosocial encounter).

We can encapsulate the modern approach to the patient–practitioner encounter by
outlining the three key factors seen in Table 1.1.

Table 1.1 Paradigm of patient-centred care: the three elements

Element	Effect	Outcome
Changes in morbidity	People living with disease and needing chronic illness management	Shifts focus from biological need to quality of life and self care
Availability of and access to medical information	Less trust in the 'paternal' system, rise in consumerism and higher patient expectations	Patients become 'experts' in their own care and treatment
Power balance towards the patient	Better-informed patient has access to medical information	Patients become active participants in their care and need information and control over their own care

What is communication?

The number of models and definitions of communication in itself signifies that communication is a vast topic and difficult to pin down to simple explanation. Communication
occurs whenever one person, in some way or another, transmits a message of some sort
and someone else picks it up and interprets it. DeVito defines communication as:

> the act, by one or more persons, of sending and receiving messages that are distorted
> by noise, occur within a context, have some effect, and provide some opportunity for
> feedback.

> (DeVito, 1988:4)

This definition implies an interaction of some kind between at least two people. It also
suggests that the interaction is two way; that the person sending the message receives
some sort of feedback, even if it is non-verbal – or even silence.

Basic models of communication have key factors in common. They usually represent a sender and a receiver of a message and some form of distortion of the message
between the sender and receiver. Such models see communication as linear, which can
be depicted in a simple flow chart (see Figure 1.2).

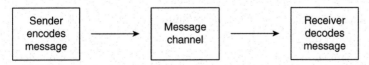

Figure 1.2 Linear model of communication

The sender needs to adapt the message in a way that can be received accurately and the receiver needs to be aware of many aspects of the sender's context, such as cognitions, culture, language and symbolism in order to decode it correctly.

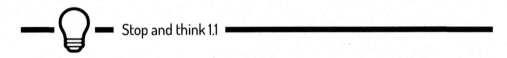

Stop and think 1.1

What is going wrong with communication in this scenario? A nurse tells a patient that the doctor is concerned about the patient's 'discharge'. The patient doesn't know if 'discharge' means a physical bodily discharge, or if the doctor is reluctant to send the patient home. See the text below for a hint.

Linear models represent the single exchange of information quite well but often do not effectively represent the complexity of the communication context and the interference, or 'noise', that is inherent in the communication process. Circular models are an attempt to convey this complexity by representing the feedback to the sender and the adjustments the sender can then make. An example is seen in Figure 1.3.

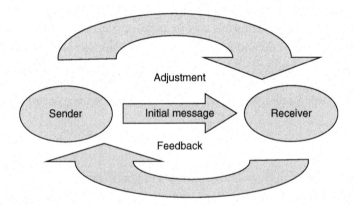

Figure 1.3   Circular model of communication

This type of model involves more than two elements of communication as the sender is also getting feedback on how the message is received. In our example in Stop and think 1.1, the patient, hearing the doctor's concern about discharge, could ask the nurse where the discharge is coming from. The nurse then adjusts her message and explains that the doctor is worried that the patient might not cope well at home.

Still, the model does not include any explanation about what has caused the misunderstanding. This is often represented in models as 'noise' or interference. A systemic model is an attempt to include this important element (see Figure 1.4).

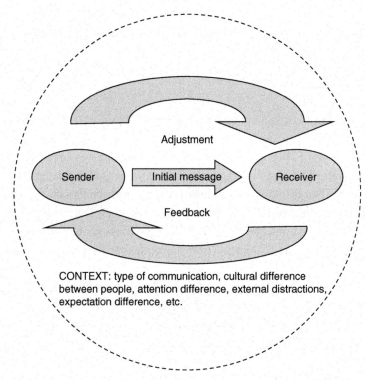

Figure 1.4 Systemic model of communication (simplified)

A systemic model acknowledges that the messages to and from the sender are subject to interference, from the very way the message in encoded, through the environmental distortions, to the way the message in decoded. A simple example might be our nurse–patient scenario of misunderstanding the word 'discharge'. The nurse assumes the patient is more aware of her condition than she actually is, and thus will understand that there is no physical discharge present. The patient, however, has not taken much notice of explanations about her condition but has been concerned about possible physical discharge after her operation; it has been on her mind, unspoken. Therefore, the patient immediately interprets the word 'discharge' to mean a physical process rather than going home.

A more complex scenario might be where a nurse is giving information to worried relatives about the condition of a loved one. The relatives may be too worried to attend to the information objectively and feel more anxious after hearing phrases that were meant to reassure, such as 'resuscitated successfully' and 'is in intensive care now'. Communication relies on a quiet and undisturbed environment with no distractions for the family or the nurse. Also, the nurse needs emotional intelligence to understand that the family are likely to be distracted and worried and require simplified language and information in order to understand accurately what the nurse says. See Practice example box 1.1.

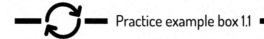

— Practice example box 1.1 —

Complex communication

A man with dementia was taken out on a trip to a steam railway. He got confused by the historical nature of the environment and refused to board the train without his wife (who had been dead some years). Rather than tell him bluntly that his wife was dead, the nurse chatted to him about events in his past, including attending a funeral with his daughter, an event he could often recall. The nurse asked him whose funeral it was and he said 'my wife's funeral'. The nurse had used a conversational approach to remind him that he was in the present and that his wife had died some time ago. To do this, the nurse needed time with the man to construct a conversation and distract him from anxiously searching for his wife and re-orient him to the present.

The man boarded the train and was appropriately sad at remembering his wife's funeral rather than distressed that she was being left behind.

Emotional intelligence

As we can see in the models and example above, effective communication relies a great deal on the ability of the message sender and the ability of the receiver to interpret the emotional content of what is being communicated.

Emotional intelligence is defined by the concept's originators as:

> the ability to perceive and express emotion, assimilate emotion in thought, understand and reason with emotion, and regulate emotion in the self and others.

(Mayer et al., 2000:396)

A growing body of evidence is demonstrating that, in nursing, the ability to relate to other people emotionally – to understand and appreciate emotional states – is key to responding in a person-centred manner and delivering more effective care. Nightingale et al. (2018) suggest that evidence for improved physical care is linked to good emotional intelligence, and Carragher and Gormley (2016) suggest that the link between emotional intelligence and good leadership leads to higher quality and compassionate care.

Knowledge link See Chapter 4 for more on emotional intelligence.

Power

Phillips (1978) describes interpersonal skills as:

> The extent to which [a person] can communicate with others, in a manner that fulfils one's rights, requirements, satisfactions, or obligations to a reasonable degree without damaging the other person's similar rights, ... in a free and open exchange.
>
> (Phillips, 1978:13)

This brings us to an important aspect of communication in healthcare: the power differential between a practitioner and a patient. Earlier, we looked at the changing nature of healthcare and used Bensing's dimensions of patient-centredness to identify the type of relationship between practitioner and patient. The history of medicine and medical practice shows how the practitioner–patient relationship was one of unequal power: the doctor was the expert and the patient was merely a recipient of their authority and learning. This describes a type of 'paternalistic' relationship of father to child. The culture of medicine and practitioner–patient relations has, arguably, retained much of this paternal structure in that the power imbalance is often still very much in favour of the practitioner. Ellis et al. (2003) suggest that power-distorted communication is common in healthcare and is embedded in the language, procedures and organisational practice that ensures domination by care professionals. Thompson (1986) suggests that, traditionally, health professionals feel better able to obtain co-operation from patients if they are in control and, when the focus of treatment is to fight the illness, the patient becomes less important in a formalised medical encounter. In such a culture, people who become patients often adopt an inferior position to the healthcare professionals and become passive recipients of care and treatment. Szasz and Hollender (1987) looked at doctor–patient relationship patterns of relating and identified three styles, outlined in Table 1.2. These can apply as much to nurses as doctors in modern healthcare, especially where nurses take a clinical lead in many aspects of care.

Table 1.2 Styles of doctor–patient relationship

Relationship style	Description	Characterised by
Activity/passivity	Full exploitation of medical power and authority	A cross-examination: doctor asks questions, patient gives answers
Guidance/co-operation	Doctor allows patient some autonomy and participation	Doctor's agenda dominates; patient is allowed some involvement within doctor's remit
Mutual participation	Both parties accept responsibility to solve problems	Patient encouraged to use the doctor's expertise to solve their health problems

Source: Szasz and Hollender, 1987

The changing nature of healthcare demands more patient empowerment in self-care and acknowledgement that the patient is often the best person to understand the context of their own healthcare management. This suggests that many nurse–patient interactions are best served by a mutual participation style of relating if the patient's long-term health and wellbeing is the objective of the healthcare professional.

It is important that nurses acknowledge power differentials inherent in patient–practitioner relationships and make the contextual and personal adjustments outlined in Figure 1.4 to facilitate communication. Burnard (1997) recognises other important power differentials that are also relevant to healthcare encounters and which may be superimposed on the pre-existing differentials, such as between people of different sex, ethnicity, culture, ability and disability, and social class. Also, for many cultures, age difference can be a source of power differential.

Nurses are expected to work in anti-oppressive and anti-discriminatory ways in accordance with the NMC *Code* requirements to respect diversity, discrimination and exclusion (NMC, 2018b). Colin Goble (2009) suggests that the nursing profession has been slower than professions such as social work to pick up on this professional requirement, perhaps because the shift from institutional to person-centred community-based care is relatively recent in nursing. However, for Goble, improved, empowering care requires nurses to develop such practice through individual and collective reflection to ensure equal access to and delivery of quality care.

Application of communication in nursing

Methods of communication

The model in Figure 1.2 suggests that the message from one person to another is encoded in some form and transmitted to the other. This encoding can involve many types of transmission format, or several types combined. For example, a person who does not want to engage in a conversation formats their information to the other by giving short answers or mumbling (vocal channels) or by reduced eye contact and folding their arms (body language). They might also try to change the subject, look at their watch (behaviour) or simply bluntly state they do not want to talk (verbal). Additionally, the communicator could write their message down or use other and more sophisticated tools for communication such as use sign language, flash cards or even a text message! DeVito (1988) states that communication is inevitable, no matter what we do; even silence or not responding says something to the other person. All behaviour, whether verbal or non-verbal, intentional or unintentional, is a form of communication, including how we move, dress, walk or use touch. As communicators, nurses need to be aware of their own intentional and unintentional messages and also be skilled in reading the messages of others.

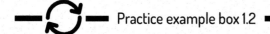 Practice example box 1.2

A reluctant patient

A shy teenage boy presenting with depression was proving to be difficult to engage in any conversation during a school visit. He had his arms and legs crossed, avoided eye contact and only gave me 'yes', 'no' and 'don't know' answers. I found I was virtually talking to the wall.

We sat in an office-cum-storage room for privacy and the room contained stacked stage and sound equipment. He frequently looked away from me at the equipment, and I read this as reluctance and discomfort in talking to me about his feelings. After some silence, I changed my focus and asked him conversationally 'what *is* all this stuff?'

He said something like 'It's stuff for school discos and so on.' He suddenly sounded confident and on surer ground so I asked him to explain what it all was. At this, he became quite animated and it appeared that he had an ambition to do DJ-ing as a hobby or career but had never had the chance to use this equipment. The conversation turned back to him and his frustrations. It was a stroke of luck that we happened to sit in that room, but no accident that I read his communication and attempted a different tack. I call this 'going fishing' when I'm with a reluctant interviewee: trying other avenues of conversation and topic to get the words flowing.

Practice example box 1.2, about a reluctant patient, shows the unintentional communication of the boy and how it was picked up by the nurse. Notice that the nurse did not know whether the change of talk would work, but that attempting to 'go through the door' that the boy was opening allowed the nurse to make a breakthrough.

DeVito also points out that communication is inevitable. When we send a message that is picked up by someone, it stays sent. We cannot unsay or negate the message, although we might need to modify its effect. Take a heated argument as an example. We've said something we later wish we hadn't said. We might then try to reduce the damage by apologising, or attempt to explain what we meant. What we are doing in fact is trying to change the message that was received. Nurses in a professional role need to maintain a professional standard of behaviour in communications with patients, relatives and colleagues, in order to maintain effective working relationships. We cannot unsay the wrong thing so it is safer to remain professional at all times until we are sure that our communication is appropriate.

Knowledge link Chapter 4 looks at channels of interpersonal communication in more detail.

The nurse–patient relationship

The relationship between the nurse and the patient is often seen as a therapeutic relationship in itself, based on partnership, intimacy and reciprocity (McMahon, 2002). Its purpose is different to a social relationship in that it has a focus on the patient's wellbeing as a priority and the nurse and patient do not need to share anything in common or even like each other (Arnold and Boggs, 2019). This relationship can last only 5 minutes in an emergency department or primary care practice, or continue and develop for months or years during chronic illness management. It can be intensely personal when breaking bad news, or quite superficial such as when directing a patient to the appropriate clinic room. However, all these scenarios are nurse–patient encounters that impart to the patient something of the support and meaningfulness of their engagement with healthcare. It tells the patient whether they are viewed as important and valued or not, whether they will be listened to or discriminated against.

+ **Knowledge link** Chapter 2 examines the nurse–patient relationship in depth.

The nurse as a member of the multi-disciplinary team

Nurses do not work with their patients in isolation. Nurses are members of multi-disciplinary teams that should co-ordinate their roles and expertise to provide the best care for patients. The NMC stipulates a level of competence in working and communicating with other health professionals in its standards for pre-registration education (NMC, 2018a). Therefore, to qualify as a nurse, students should be able to contribute to team working by understanding their own role in the team, respecting the roles of others and managing the resources available within the team for the benefit of their patients. Working with others from different professional backgrounds, often with different priorities, can be challenging but it is often the nurse who takes the lead in co-ordinating health-based care by using good communication and management skills.

+ **Knowledge link** Chapter 5 will explore working in groups and teams in more depth.

Conclusion

This book is intended for nurses, nursing associates and apprentices in education and training as well as newly qualified nurses. Chapters are written to apply to all fields of care and strive to address the needs of all or any nurse in a range of settings.

Some practice examples given in the chapters may appear to be specific to one particular field of care, for example, a case study in the emergency department, or working with children. However, each scenario can be applied across a range of practice areas and the communication skills being addressed are applicable to all fields of care. Therefore, each chapter has something to offer nurse students pursuing any particular care area.

It is recognised that different fields of nursing care may use different terminology for patients, carers, service users and so on. In the main we have chosen to refer to recipients of direct care as patients. Some areas of care use the term client to refer to the person being cared for, and so you will also see that term used in the book. Family members or informal carers are referred to as carers. We have also used the terms children and young people to differentiate younger children from adolescents, as the needs of these two age groups can often be very different according to their psychological and social developmental stages.

Also, we have attempted to make clear that references to patients, family members and nurses in general that are not gender specific by referring to these groups as 'they' singular. However, some authors may refer to a nurse as gendered because the author is self-identifying with the nurse.

FURTHER READING

Burnard, P. and Gill, P. (2013) *Culture, Communication and Nursing*. London, Routledge.
McCray, J. (ed.) (2009) *Nursing and Multi-professional Practice*. London, SAGE Publications.

REFERENCES

Arnold, E. and Boggs, K. (2019) *Interpersonal Relationships: Professional Communication Skills for Nurses* (8th edn). London, Elsevier.
Bensing, J. (2000) Bridging the gap: the separate worlds of evidence-based medicine and patient-centred medicine. *Patient Education and Counseling*, 39, 17–25.
Bensing, J.M. and Verheul, W. (2010) The silent healer: the role of communication in placebo effects. *Patient Education and Counseling*, 80(3), 293–299.
Burnard, P. (1997) *Effective Communication Skills for Health Professionals* (2nd edn). Cheltenham, Stanley Thornes.
Carragher, J. and Gormley, K. (2017) Leadership and emotional intelligence in nursing and midwifery education and practice: a discussion paper. *Journal of Advanced Nursing*, 73(1), 85–96. doi: 10.1111/jan.13141.
DeVito, J. (1988) *Human Communication: The Basic Course*. New York, Harper & Row.
Ellis, R., Gates, B. and Kenworthy, N. (2003) *Interpersonal Communication in Nursing: Theory and Practice*. Edinburgh, Churchill Livingstone.
Fitzpatrick, L. (2018) The importance of communication and professional values relating to nursing practice. *Links to Health and Social Care*, 3(1), 26–40.

Goble, C. (2009) Multi-professional working in the community. In J. McCray (ed.), *Nursing and Multi-professional Practice* (pp. 49–65). London, SAGE Publications.

Mayer, J.D., Salovey, P. and Caruso, D.R. (2000) Models of emotional intelligence. In R.J. Sternberg (ed.), *Handbook of Intelligence* (pp. 396–420). New York, Cambridge University Press.

McMahon, R. (2002) Therapeutic nursing: theory, issues and practice. In R. McMahon and A. Pearson (eds), *Nursing as Therapy* (p. 1). Cheltenham, Nelson Thornes.

Nightingale, S., Spiby, H., Kayleigh, S. and Sladen, P. (2018) The impact of emotional intelligence in health care professionals on caring behaviour towards patients in clinical and long-term care settings: findings from an integrative review. *International Journal of Nursing Studies*, 80, 106–117. doi: 10.1016/j.ijnurstu.2018.01.006.

NMC (2018a) *Future Nurse: Standards of Proficiency for Registered Nurses.* www.nmc.org.uk/globalassets/sitedocuments/education-standards/future-nurse-proficiencies.pdf.

NMC (2018b) *The Code: Professional Standards of Practice and Behaviour for Nurses, Midwives and Nursing Associates.* www.nmc.org.uk/standards/code/.

Ogden, J. (2012) *Health Psychology: A Textbook* (5th edn). Buckingham, Open University Press.

Phillips, E. (1978) *The Social Skills Basis of Psychopathology.* New York, Grune & Stratton.

Popa-Velea, O. and Purcărea, V.L. (2014) Issues of therapeutic communication relevant for improving quality of care. *Journal of Medicine and Life*, 7(S4), 39–45.

Raghubir, A. (2018) Emotional intelligence in professional nursing practice: a concept review using Rodgers's evolutionary analysis approach. *International Journal of Nursing Sciences*, 5, 126–130.

RCN (2018) *Principles of Nursing Practice.* www.rcn.org.uk/professional-development/principles-of-nursing-practice.

Street, R., Makoul, G., Arora, N. and Epstein, R. (2009) How does communication heal? Pathways linking clinician–patient communication to health outcomes. *Patient Education and Counseling*, 74, 295–301.

Szasz, T.S. and Hollender, M.H. (1956) A contribution to the philosophy of medicine: the basic models of the doctor-patient relationship. *AMA Archives of Internal Medicine*, 97(5), 585–592.

TWO
THE NURSE–PATIENT RELATIONSHIP
EULA MILLER AND GAYATRI NAMBIAR-GREENWOOD

....THIS CHAPTER WILL HELP YOU TO:

- Engage with people to build professional relationships
- Recognise barriers to developing effective relationships
- Initiate, maintain and close professional relationships
- Develop self-awareness and challenge your own prejudices

Introduction

The nurse–patient relationship is central to meeting the patient's care needs and communication between the nurse and patient is the foundation on which this relationship is built (Kourkouta and Papathanasiou, 2014; Arnold and Boggs, 2015). According to Ha and Longnecker (2010), patients value the uncomplicated style of interaction, continuity of care and nurse–patient time, all of which are afforded by the nurse–patient relationship.

The UK National Health Service (NHS) statutory guidance on involving people in their own health and care (NHS, 2017) recommends that healthcare professionals should value, respect and listen to service users as individuals. For the purposes of this chapter, the nurse–patient relationship is defined as a series of planned interactions that have the patient's need at their core. These interventions focus on the feelings, priorities, challenges and ideas of the patient, with the progressive aim of enhancing optimum physical, spiritual and mental health. The nurse–patient relationship is, therefore, based on patient-centred nursing, which is only possible when there is solid and reliable communication between nurse and patient.

However, there are inherent inequalities in the nurse–patient relationship (Ozaras and Abaan, 2018). Unlike social relationships, patients have little choice about the health professionals who will care for them. This powerlessness renders the patient vulnerable, and makes them reliant and dependent on practitioners for effectively intervening in their care (Sheridan et al., 2015). The nurse then has a responsibility to interact, educate and share information that genuinely has the patient's best interest central to the delivery of care (NMC, 2018). The development and management of an effective nurse–patient relationship is therefore a key skill in nursing, in any field of care.

The foundation of therapeutic relationships

Self-awareness

The first step to being able to facilitate effective communication is **self-awareness**. An individual cannot understand others until they come to know themselves. This concept has been documented in nursing literature for a number of decades (Boud et al., 1985; Burnard, 1992; Freshwater, 2002; Jack and Smith, 2007; Rasheed, 2015). Self-awareness allows us to relate to the experience of others, while developing the essential skill of empathy. It commences from early childhood when we are first able to recognise ourselves in a mirror (around 18 months–2 years old), and continues throughout our life.

Healey and McSharry (2011) suggest that a nurse requires the ability to think, feel and act appropriately in order to develop skills of self-awareness. Therefore, for example, if a nurse has not come to terms with a personal bereavement, they may cope less effectively with the needs of a dying patient because of the fears and discomforts the episode can generate.

There are a number of useful tools that promote self-awareness, for example the Johari window (Table 2.1).

Table 2.1   The Johari window

	Known to self	Not known to self
Known to others	Open area	Blind area
Not known others	Hidden area	Unknown area

Source: Luft, 1969

The Johari window is a well-known model of the self that can be used as a tool for mapping development of self-awareness. It is named after its constructors, Joe Luft and Harry Ingham (Gill et al., 2015). The model challenges us to reflect on and explore aspects of ourselves that we may rarely consider normally. To explore and expand our knowledge of each window, we can set ourselves tasks of self-reflection or feedback from others.

The open area is what we present to others and what is observed by others. This can be dominated by 'false fronts' or 'masks' that we present to the world and perhaps ourselves, or aspects of ourselves we are comfortable to share with others, such as our confidence or shyness. The hidden area contains those aspects we know about but don't want to share, perhaps anger or jealousy. The blind area is those aspects others detect about us but of which we are personally unaware. This area is often best explored through feedback from other people. The unknown area is that which is hidden even from ourselves, and too painful to confront or bring to consciousness. Personal development in self-awareness will make the open and hidden windows bigger and the blind and unknown windows smaller.

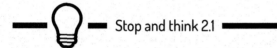 Stop and think 2.1

Think of at least five aspects of yourself (what makes you, *you*) that apply to the open and hidden areas. You could put a copy of this in your portfolio and add to it throughout your course of study. As you gain different experiences in practice settings, you will be able to demonstrate self-awareness development by entering what you discover about yourself as a nurse in the blind and unknown areas. You can even record in your portfolio how you discovered these things about yourself.

Jack and Miller (2008) documented a more recent adaptation to this self-awareness tool, specifically developed for nurses. These authors refer to it as the Self-Development Awareness Tool (Box 2.1).

The tool is divided into three stages of interpersonal acquisition, which are the Now stage, followed by the Transitional stage and finally the Re-group stage. Box 2.1 shows tool's intricacies and the cue questions set at each stage that potentially facilitate the nurse's journey to becoming more self-aware.

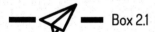 Box 2.1

The Self-Development Awareness Tool (Jack and Miller, 2008)

The Now stage:

- Who am I at this moment? (Taking into account thoughts, feelings and behaviour.)
- What do I know about myself and what do I show to others? (Past experiences may dictate how we behave. Contextual influences such as the behaviour of others in the practice setting may have an influence on this.)
- What is it I would like to be more aware of? (This can be difficult but try to imagine how others see you. They may be aware of certain behaviours that you had not even thought about.)

(Continued)

- What has triggered this desire to change? (Consider what it is you feel uncomfortable about, or what it is you would like to develop. It may be that certain assumptions you have are holding you back. Your motivation may be a personal desire to be more assertive with others, for example.)

The Transition stage:

- What strengths/limitations do I have already? (This will require a certain amount of honesty.)
- What do I need to develop? (You may need to seek support from others. This is a proactive process as you actively engage in and develop new learning to inform practice.)
- What are the opportunities and threats to my development? (You may need to discard prior experiences if they are causing conflict and build on more positive experiences that you have been part of.)

The Re-group stage:

- Where am I now? (What new knowledge have I gained about myself and the situation?)
- What has changed about me and the way I am in this situation? (Do I now think, feel and engage in a different way in these situations?)
- How do we grow/where do we go from here? (How can we develop this new learning and way of being?)
- Acceptance of self at this stage.

The experience of this journey should affect our delivery of practice as we are able to recognise our strengths and limitations and an appreciation for our own acts and omissions in the care of those who require our help.

Empathy

Reynolds (2017) suggests that empathy is the capacity to enter or view the lived experience of the other person. It is easy for the new student nurse to confuse sympathy with empathy; however, the difference is fundamental. Sympathy is relating to another as though they were us and we were experiencing their situation. Empathy can be differentiated as being able to relate to another directly and understand how *they* experience their situation.

Sympathy is the ability to put ourselves in someone else's shoes: 'If that were me, I'd be very upset.'

Empathy is the ability to be in someone else's shoes. 'I can sense you were very upset.'

Empathy in practice also needs to be demonstrated to the other person to convey support and understanding and to be able to share the other's experience. This is done by communication! See Box 2.2 for the view of a trained hostage negotiator.

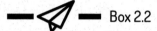 **Box 2.2**

The hostage negotiator's view of empathy

A trained hostage negotiator claims that the key communication skill essential for gaining trust and engagement in the negotiation process is empathy. A good negotiator may be there for the hostages, but needs to understand the position of the hostage takers. So, a good negotiator has sympathy for the hostages, but empathy for the hostage takers (Dawson, 2010).

Trust

A nurse–patient relationship is based on trust. The patient needs to feel able to disclose personal and possibly painful information about themselves and ask questions that require courage to voice. If a patient cannot ask a nurse a question that begins with, 'I know this is going to sound silly, but ...', who can they ask?

For this reason, the NMC *Code* (NMC, 2018) insists that nurses demonstrate respect for patients, ensuring and protecting the dignity and confidentiality of patients. A registered nurse must at all times uphold public trust in the nursing profession (NMC, 2018).

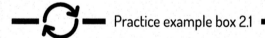 **Practice example box 2.1**

Confidentiality

An off-duty registered nurse on a train overheard three young women, obviously student nurses, discussing a patient from their recent practice experience. They commented on his appearance, behaviour and his family, in derogatory terms. They named the ward he was on and discussed how they would try to avoid him in future. This conversation could be overheard by all passengers in the vicinity. The registered nurse reminded the students of the *Code* (NMC, 2018) and pointed out that the general public would not be happy to be nursed by people who would discuss them in such a way.

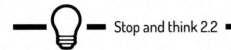 **Stop and think 2.2**

Consider what essential qualities you would expect in someone nursing you or a loved one. Do you measure up to those expectations? What skills and personal qualities do you need to develop to become such a nurse? What qualities do you have already? Have they been recorded in your Johari window?

Your portfolio Johari window will now become historical: what you put in to your blind and unknown areas will be those things you did not know about yourself but have since discovered during your nursing practice. The Johari window in your portfolio will act as evidence of your personal and professional development in self-awareness and communication skills.

Non-judgemental relating

The *Code* (NMC, 2018) demands that nurses offer fair and equal care to patients from diverse backgrounds and circumstances. Nurses are not expected to be saints or have no opinions of their own, but, as a nurse, in whatever circumstances, we need to put aside personal opinions in order to offer the best care we can. We do not have to agree with the values, opinions or behaviour of our patients outside the health context. However, we have to be able to accept the person for who they are regardless of differences in morals, beliefs and behaviours.

As a nurse, we could be caring for a patient who has been transferred from prison while serving time for some heinous crime, but such patients still have heart attacks, strokes or get depressed. Equally, we might want to 'go the extra mile' for someone we particularly like, but need to be mindful of what is appropriate. The nurse–patient relationship is a professional one that respects the patient in their health context regardless of our personal views.

Genuineness and authenticity

It would be difficult to develop trust in our patients if professionally we were not trustworthy or genuinely interested in their welfare. It is sometimes difficult to empathise with a person's situation when their behaviour or attitude is very different from our own. **Genuineness** refers to being the authentic self that we present to the patient; being kind because we are kind, being interested because we are interested. This is acting with **authenticity**. Genuineness is suggested by Rogers (1967) to be a core principle in developing a therapeutic relationship. However, this is not without its challenges. Nurses are expected to improve a patient's way of life towards health. As such, the more a nurse is able to act with authenticity in their professional relationships while being able to be empathetic, trustworthy and non-judgemental, the higher the quality of care such a nurse is likely to achieve. Genuineness is a fundamental quality of nursing practice. Becoming authentic in our practice requires us to work on our professional development.

The nurse–patient relationship must commence, develop and terminate with the patient being confident that their nurse understands their situation, respects them as an individual and does not judge them, but is someone who can invest time and interest in their wellbeing.

Boundaries

The NMC describes **boundaries** as defining:

> the limits of behaviour which allow a nurse or midwife to have a professional relationship with the person in their care.
>
> (NMC, 2008:1)

We can regard the nurse–patient relationship as a process that has goals. It aims to be therapeutic (good for the patient) and facilitative (enabling nursing care). We could add **humanistic**, in that it also aims to be positive, **beneficent** to all concerned and non-harmful (**non-maleficent**) to either the patient or the nurse. It is important to recognise that the nurse is not expected to be wholly self-sacrificial in their relationships with patients. There is no room, for example, for nurses to be abused or exploited by patients outside the context of their illness. Nurses should not suffer physical or verbal injury in their role, although patients can and often do express their hurt and anger to their nurses.

However, as noted in Chapter 1, the nurse–patient relationship involves a power differential in favour of the nurse. For the NMC (2018), nurses carry the responsibility to maintain appropriate boundaries to the relationship with their patient, and conducting personal relationships with vulnerable patients is never acceptable.

Practice example box 2.2 was used by the UK Central Council (UKCC; now the NMC) to illustrate financial abuse.

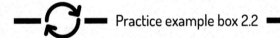 Practice example box 2.2

Example of a breach of boundaries

Chloe nursed Miss G in her own home. Miss G was paralysed following a bout of meningitis 2 years ago. Although she required total physical care, she could write her name. During the 6 months in which Chloe had cared for her, Miss G had loaned her a total of £200. Chloe had told Miss G that she could not cope on her salary as an agency staff nurse.

(UKCC, 1999:6)

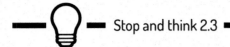 **Stop and think 2.3**

Look at Practice example box 2.2. What professional issues do you think this example raises? The answers from the UKCC are listed here. The UKCC outlined the following professional issues raised by the example:

- The vulnerability and dependency of Miss G
- The imbalance of power in the relationship
- Miss G's fear of the withdrawal of care is she does not agree to lend the nurse, Chloe, money
- Intimidation and exploitation of the patient, even if it is unintentional
- The distortion of the boundaries to the professional practitioner–patient relationship
- Moving the focus of care away from meeting the patient's needs towards meeting the practitioner's own needs
- Financial abuse covers the inappropriate use of a patient's funds, property or resources and this includes borrowing money from a patient.

The example in Practice example box 2.2 illustrates how the blurring of the professional and personal boundaries can result in abuse of the patient. The professional relationship often necessarily involves intimacy between the nurse and the patient, but generally personal and intimate information should pass from the patient to the nurse, not the other way around. However, there is some place for sharing personal information in order to convey empathy and understanding. The nurse is required to know what is appropriate and must be guided by ensuring that their care relationship is based on public trust in the profession.

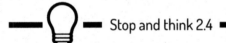 **Stop and think 2.4**

Cover up the central and right-hand columns on the list of behaviours shown in Table 2.2 and decide whether each behaviour would be acceptable in *any* nurse–patient relationship. Remember, this could apply to short- or long-term relationships with surgical, medical adult patients, children and their families, or adults or children with learning difficulties or mental illness. See if you agree with the advice given.

Table 2.2 Nursing boundaries

Behaviour	Answer	Rationale
Beginning a personal relationship with an ex-patient immediately after treatment/discharge	No	Not *immediately* after a relationship and certainly not if the person is in any way still in a dependent and vulnerable state. The nurse's knowledge of the person has been gained from a privileged position.

Visiting a person's home unannounced and without an appointment	No	Unless in an emergency where there are serious concerns about safety of the patient or others in their care.
Seeing a person in your care outside your normal practice hours	No	There should be no need to work outside normal practice hours. If the patient needs this they should be referred to the appropriate service.
Lending a patient money	No	Under any circumstances
Borrowing money from a patient	No	Under any circumstances
Commencing a sexual relationship with a patient's relative	No	The relative is also in a vulnerable position and the relationship will additionally affect the nurse–patient relationship.
Buying a car from a patient	No	This blurs the boundaries between a professional and social/ business relationship.
Telling 'dirty' jokes	No	There is a danger of this being interpreted as sexual harassment or flirtatious behaviour from the nurse, and is, by definition, over-familiarity.
Discussing sexual matters not relevant to care or treatment	No	As above. This might apply to health promotion or aiding personal development, but should have solely a care aim and be part of the care plan.
Allowing a patient to repeatedly hit you because they are frustrated/angry	No	Some might regard this as 'cathartic' in allowing the patient to express their feelings. However, the other message this conveys is that hitting the carer is appropriate. This might be 'tolerated' on occasion, but never 'allowed' or encouraged.
Referring a patient to a colleague because the patient makes persistent sexual references about you	Yes	If the therapeutic relationship is in danger of breaking down because of a patient's behaviour or misunderstanding it is appropriate to recognise your limitations and facilitate a safer professional relationship.

If you are unsure of any of these answers, make it an action point for your next practice placement and discuss a range of scenarios with your practice facilitator. There are very few exceptions to these general guidelines but the skill of the qualified nurse is deciding how to justify such exceptions in the context of a patient's care. Remember, the nurse–patient relationship necessarily incorporates a power imbalance, rendering the patient vulnerable and dependent on their nurse. It is the responsibility of the nurse to maintain the professional division between patient and nurse and resist attempts from the patient to blur these boundaries. In so doing, the nurse can optimise the delivery of effective care.

Knowledge link There is more on therapeutic relationships in Chapter 4.

The nurse–patient relationship process

The nurse–patient relationship can be described as a good story: it has a beginning, a middle and an end. Even in a very short or long relationship, the basic pattern should be the same. We make contact with patients for the first time and commence the relationship-building process. Then we use the relationship to deliver care and, finally, we complete the relationship by ensuring the patient is no longer dependent on us and ready to 'move on'. This process is described variously in nursing and other therapeutic health professions, but frequently in the similar terms of a staged process. Below we will look at two of these.

Peplau's developmental model: a nursing model of the nurse–patient relationship

Peplau (1997) suggested that the nurse–patient relationship can be divided into four phases, and that the nurse may have a range of roles to play within the relationship. See Table 2.3.

Table 2.3   The four phases of the nurse–patient relationship

Phase	For the patient	For the nurse
1 Orientation	The person seeks professional assistance	The patient's needs are unknown. Establish a rapport and assist patient in developing a working relationship.
2 Identification	The patient uses the nurse to find out what the problems are	Encourage person to identify health problems and express feelings about them.
3 Exploitation	The patient makes use of the nurse to problem-solve	Develop the patient's competencies and facilitate person's recovery and development. Act as a healthcare resource and facilitate external resources.
4 Resolution	The person becomes freed of the need for help from the nurse	Goal set for person's future. Facilitate independence and self-care. Withdraw when no longer needed.

Source: Peplau, 1997

For Peplau, the nurse acts as a stranger (in the orientation phase), then as a resource, leader, surrogate and counsellor (in the other three phases). Peplau's model can be seen as patient-centred and the nurse takes on a facilitative role rather than setting the agenda. Perhaps unlike Roper, Logan and Tierney's model (Holland et al., 2008), where the patient's needs are determined by a pre-set list of factors (the Activities of Daily Living), Peplau's model depends on the nurse and patient identifying the patient's needs together. Arguably, Peplau's model is therefore more patient-centred.

Burnard's eight-stage counselling map

Burnard (2005) suggests a similar process suitable for counselling but also reflects the patient-centred approach (Table 2.4).

Table 2.4 Summary of Burnard's eight-stage counselling map

Stage	Counselling goals	Possible nursing practice
1	Meeting and establishing 'boundaries'	Introduction and initial assessment; relationship commencement
2	Discussing surface issues, testing safety, engagement	Getting to know each other, discussing routine health issues and surface health context of personal issues
3	Deeper issues: disclosures on deeper levels and using trust	Exploring person's healthcare concerns, identifying holistic needs and gaps in self-care
4	Ownership of feelings – cathartic	Encouraging person to address their relationship with health issues, i.e. heart disease fears or medication side effects
5	Developing client's insight and problem identification	Seeking and encouraging person's response to health information and self-statements of hopes, fears ideas for coping and barriers to health, i.e., 'I'm too stressed all the time, I shouldn't work so hard'
6	Exploration of problems and possible solutions	Discussion of identified problems, and encouraging person to find and 'own' solutions, i.e. 'I shall have to cut down my hours while I recover'
7	Client action and practitioner support	Giving attention and support to person's new health behaviour: motivating, educating, facilitating resources
8	Disengagement and management of 'letting go' anxieties	Empowering person to continue without you, finding more appropriate support, considering the future without the nurse–patient relationship

Source: Burnard, 2005:119–126

Burnard's stages consider the counselling aspect of the practitioner–patient relationship, but can be applied to the nurse's role as an advocate and as a hands-on carer. Whether the patient is depressed, has developed a chronic health problem such as diabetes or schizophrenia, or is having straightforward elective surgery, the nurse helps the patient to explore their health beliefs, attitudes, knowledge or behaviour. In doing this, the nurse's role is using the nurse–patient relationship to enhance the patient's relationship with their health problem.

Conclusion

This chapter has focused on defining the nurse–patient relationship rather than techniques to establish and manage an effective relationship. It has addressed some of the issues of managing boundaries, but mainly aims to define a good relationship and what may constitute a breakdown of the professional therapeutic space between nurse and patient. Management of a good nurse–patient relationship relies on some key personal and professional skills. These skills are largely good self-awareness of our own motivations, values and characteristics, together with personal qualities such as approachability and trustworthiness. These factors are underpinned by good skills in leading the relationship and understanding its objectives.

The nurse–patient relationship underpins all our encounters with patients and other service users. Without a sound understanding of and ability to engage in a nurse–patient relationship, we cannot deliver effective patient-centred care.

REFERENCES

Arnold, E.C. and Boggs, K.U. (2015) *Interpersonal Relationships: Professional Communication Skills for Nurses*. St. Louis, MI, Elsevier.

Boud, D., Keogh, R. and Walker, D. (1985) *Reflection: Turning Experience into Learning*. London, Kogan Page.

Burnard, P. (1992) *Know Yourself: Self Awareness Activities for Nurses*. London, Scutari.

Burnard, P. (2005) *Counselling Skills for Health Professionals* (4th edn). Cheltenham, Nelson Thornes.

Dawson, K. (2010) *Thank you for my Freedom* (radio broadcast). Whistledown Productions. Originally available on www.bbc.co.uk/programmes/b00s2yll.

Freshwater, D. (ed.) (2002) *Therapeutic Nursing*. London, SAGE Publications.

Gill, L.J., Ramsey, P.L. and Leberman, S.I. (2015) A systems approach to developing emotional intelligence using the self-awareness engine of growth model. *Systemic Practice and Action Research*, 28(6), 575–594.

Ha, J.F. and Longnecker, N. (2010) Doctor-patient communication: a review. *The Ochsner Journal*, 10(1), 38–43.

Healy, D. and McSharry, P. (2011) Promoting self-awareness in undergraduate nursing students in relation to their health status and personal behaviours. *Nurse Education in Practice*, 11(4), 228–233.

Holland, K., Jenkins, J., Solomon, J. and Whittam, S. (2008) *Applying the Roper, Logan & Tierney Model in Practice* (2nd edn). Edinburgh, Elsevier.

Jack, K. and Smith, A. (2007) Promoting self-awareness in nurses to improve nursing practice. *Nursing Standard*, 21(32), 47–52.

Jack, K. and Miller, E. (2008) Exploring self-awareness in mental health practice. *Mental Health Practice*, 12(3), 31–35.

Kourkouta, L. and Papathanasiou, I.V. (2014) Communication in nursing practice. *Materia Socio-Medica*, 26(1), 65.

Luft, J. (1969) *Of Human Interaction*. Palo Alto, CA, National Press Books.

NHS (2017) *Involving People in Their Own Health and Care (Statutory Guidance)*. www.england. nhs.uk/commissioning/wp-content/uploads/sites/12/2015/10/ohc-paper-06.pdf.

NMC (2008) *The Code: Standards of Conduct, Performance and Ethics for Nurses and Midwives*. London, Nursing and Midwifery Council.

NMC (2018) *The Code: Professional Standards of Practice and Behaviour for Nurses, Midwives and Nursing Associates*. www.nmc.org.uk/standards/code/.

Ozaras, G. and Abaan, S. (2018) Investigation of the trust status of the nurse–patient relationship. *Nursing Ethics*, 25(5), 628–639.

Peplau, H.E. (1997) Peplau's theory of interpersonal relations. *Nursing Science Quarterly*, 10(4), 162–167.

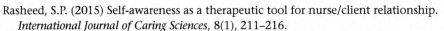

Rasheed, S.P. (2015) Self-awareness as a therapeutic tool for nurse/client relationship. *International Journal of Caring Sciences*, 8(1), 211–216.

Reynolds, W.J. (2017) *The Measurement and Development of Empathy in Nursing*. London, Routledge.

Rogers, C. (1967) *On Becoming a Person: A Therapist's View of Psychotherapy*. London, Constable.

Sheridan, N.F., Kenealy, T.W., Kidd, J.D., Schmidt-Busby, J.I., Hand, J.E., Raphael, D.L. and Rea, H.H. (2015) Patients' engagement in primary care: powerlessness and compounding jeopardy: a qualitative study. *Health Expectations*, 18(1), 32–43.

UKCC (1999) Nurses, midwives and health visitors must maintain proper boundaries to relationships with patients and clients. *Register*, 29, 6–7.

THREE
HOW TO RELATE TO OTHERS EFFECTIVELY

LUCY WEBB

.... THIS CHAPTER WILL HELP YOU TO:

- Engage with people and build caring professional relationships
- Recognise and overcome barriers in developing relationships with patients
- Develop self-awareness and challenge your own prejudices
- Use helpful and therapeutic strategies to enable people to understand treatments and give informed consent
- Work confidently as part of a team
- Work with people to provide clear and accurate information

Introduction

In this chapter we will explore two different ways of relating to others that help the nurse establish trust, confidence and co-operation from others.

When we talk to friends and family, we relate to them on the basis of our existing relationships. For instance, we can be relaxed and playful with brothers and sisters, dependent on parents and partners, trusting with friends and perhaps authoritative with children. When we don't know someone very well, we make assumptions about how we should relate to them; for example, 'They seem shy, I'll do all the talking!'

As a nurse, you will meet a lot of patients with different needs and personal characteristics. You must be able to relate to them in way that is professionally appropriate and enables you to develop a good working relationship with each person you meet. For instance, that shy patient needs to be encouraged to talk so that you can find out something important about their health worries. Knowing when to 'do all the talking' and when to 'do the listening' is a key skill in communication. This chapter will help you develop skills in *when* to listen or talk, and *how* to listen and talk.

There are some useful models of communication and relationships that help us understand how we need to present ourselves to others and how to understand someone by their way of communicating. In this chapter, we will look at two common models used in nursing. The first half of the chapter we will look at transactional analysis and in the second half we'll look at six-category intervention analysis.

Transactional analysis

Transactional analysis (or **TA**) is a model of communication developed by Eric Berne (1964). It helps professionals understand what effect their style of communication has on others and how to develop more effective communication. Transactional analysis is one of the most common communication skills models used in nursing and has several different components, which are outlined below.

Ego states

An **ego state** could be described as the self-concept or attitude of mind or 'role' a person adopts when communicating with others. Berne (1964) identified three ego states: parent, adult and child.

In the example below, a nurse is talking to an anxious patient about her operation:

Nurse: 'Now, Jane, there's nothing to worry about. It's only a minor operation and you'll be awake and right as rain in no time.'

What age difference is there between these two people, do you think? Is Jane an adult or a child? Does the nurse sound like an adult, a parent or a child? Now look at the same scenario acted out below.

Nurse: 'I can see you're anxious about this operation. What can I do to reassure you?'

What's the difference? Which do you think is better? We could say that the difference is the attitude of mind the nurse has taken with the patient. In the first example the nurse is a parent figure taking an authoritative position over the patient. In the second, the nurse has taken a position of equality and spoken to the patient as one adult to another. Which is better can depend on the patient's needs and the nursing outcome desired. One type of ego state can make the other person adopt a reciprocal state. Look at the next example of an exchange between a nurse tutor and a student nurse:

Tutor: 'If you continue to turn up late for tutorials, I can't be expected to wait around for you. I will have to see someone else in your place.'

Student: 'But I live further away than most people and have to rely on the bus. It's not fair.'

The tutor is adopting a parent ego state and has elicited a child ego state in response. See Figure 3.1.

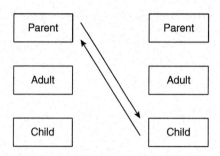

Figure 3.1 A classic ego state of parent and child

In transactional analysis, an ego state can be like a parent, adult or child. A parent state can be caring (a **nurturing parent**) or judgemental or authoritarian (a **critical parent**). A child state can be happy and carefree (a **natural child**), or sulky, stubborn, compliant or rebellious (an **adapted child**). See Box 3.1 for an example of each state.

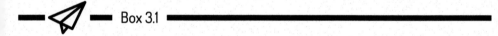 Box 3.1

Ego states and sub-states

Nurturing parent: 'It will all be better soon.'
Critical parent: 'You missed your appointment time. You'll just have to wait at the end.'
Adapted child: 'I don't see why I have to wait! There's no one else here!'
Natural child: 'I don't mind. I've nothing better to do!'

Strokes

When we communicate with someone, we give them attention. Berne called these attention episodes **strokes**. Strokes can be either positive or negative depending on whether we mean to be encouraging or discouraging. Bullying would be a good example of negative stroking, while praise would be positive stroking.

Positive strokes give approval, encouragement, praise or affection and improve another's self-esteem and confidence.

Negative strokes communicate disapproval and dislike, and give rise to a person avoiding further contacts and communication, losing confidence and developing low self-esteem.

Look at the transactions below and note the negative or positive stroking and the ego states adopted.

Example 3.1: Father to his child (Figure 3.2)

Father: 'You'll never do it that way. You've got it all wrong!'

Small child (knocking over bricks deliberately): 'It's stupid anyway.'

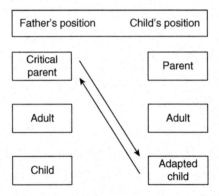

Figure 3.2 Interaction of critical parent and adapted child

Example 3.2: Ward sister to student nurse (Figure 3.3)

Sister: 'There, you see? You can give injections properly. It's just a matter of practice.'

Student nurse: 'Oh, it's easy isn't it? Now I've got the hang of it I'll do them all now!'

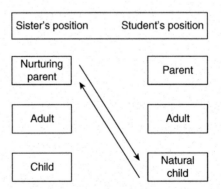

Figure 3.3 Interaction of nurturing parent and natural child

Example 3.3: Student nurse to patient (Figure 3.4)

Student nurse: 'I'm afraid there will be a bit of a wait. Would you like some tea or anything?'

Patient: 'That's alright nurse. I've got a magazine to read. I'll just wait.'

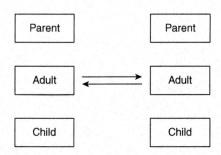

Figure 3.4   Adult-to-adult interaction

In Example 3.1, the father adopts a critical parent ego state and gives his child a negative stroke by criticising the child's attempts to build something with bricks. The child is discouraged and responds by adopting a rebellious adapted child ego state. Imagine what a childhood spent receiving a lot of negative strokes like this would do to a child's confidence and self-esteem as they grow up.

In Example 3.2, the ward sister is a nurturing parent by giving praise for performing a skill successfully. This is accepted by the student who, feeling more confident about the skill, jokes about her enthusiasm. In this way the student adopts a natural child ego state.

In Example 3.3 you may have spotted that the student nurse communicates information to the patient in a manner of equality and respect for the other's ability to make decisions. This is adult-to-adult relating and the patient responds in an appropriate adult way.

Transactions

The examples above also demonstrate that, in a communication **transaction**, one ego state can elicit a corresponding ego state. The critical parent state elicits an adapted child, the nurturing parent elicits a natural child and the adult ego state of the student nurse elicits an adult ego state response from the patient. We respond to another's ego state by adopting what is appropriate, or what our egos need, for the situation. We can also use a particular ego state to deliberately elicit a desired ego state. Look at the examples below.

Example 3.4: Ward sister to nurse

A ward sister comes into the laundry storeroom where a newly qualified staff nurse and a healthcare assistant are sorting out the fresh laundry. It is time for the handover and the sister wants the staff nurse to attend on time.

Sister:	'Do hurry up with that laundry, nurse! Everyone is waiting for you!'
Nurse:	'I can't do it any faster!'
[Sister leaves] Nurse to healthcare assistant:	'She got out of the wrong side of bed this morning.'
Healthcare assistant:	'Yeah, probably fell out!'

The sister starts as a critical parent and the nurse responds as an adapted child. The sister may have felt annoyed and so gave out a negative stroke to make herself feel better and the nurse responded defensively to it. The nurse then adopts a natural child with the healthcare assistant in order to gain an ally (and a positive stroke). The healthcare assistant obliges by also adopting a natural child ego state and gives the desired positive stroke.

The dynamics of this team suggest a division between the leadership and others that is likely to lead to communication avoidance, lack of trust in the leader and lack of responsibility from the team. The ward sister is seen as a critical parent and the team become irresponsible children as they adopt child ego states with the sister and each other.

A better approach from the sister might be as follows.

Sister:	'Handover is about to start. It's important that you're present at the beginning for this one.'
Nurse:	'OK, sister. I'll be there on time.'
[Sister leaves] Nurse to healthcare assistant:	'I'd better do this later or I'll be late for handover.'
Healthcare assistant:	'That's OK, I'll manage this myself. You go.'

In this example, the sister adopts an adult ego state, and the nurse responds also with an adult ego state. The nurse does not need to be defensive or look for an ally elsewhere. The nurse can then relate to the healthcare assistant with an adult-to-adult transaction and elicits an adult ego state response.

This dynamic would suggest that this team respect each other's roles, and can communicate unwelcome information effectively and without putting others down. This team treat each other as responsible adults and this probably works with patients too!

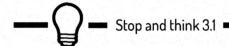

Stop and think 3.1

When you are next on placement or in a social setting, observe the communication between people and try to identify the transactions taking place.

Check with your mentor by relating your observations and see if they agree with you. This is also a skills development exercise in reflection and supervision.

Crossed transactions

When communication goes wrong, we can often see a crossed transaction where one person has misinterpreted the ego state of the other. See Box 3.2.

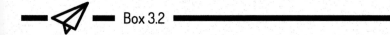

Box 3.2

A crossed transaction

In a pre-operation clinic an anxious patient asks the doctor what the risks are. The doctor responds by giving a detailed description of the procedure. The patient gets more anxious and refuses to sign the consent form.

This patient was anxious and probably in an adapted child ego state, trying to elicit reassurance in a controlled way. The doctor, however, responded in an adult ego state and didn't give the needed reassurance (Figure 3.5). A nurturing parent ego state from the doctor would have been more appropriate in the circumstances.

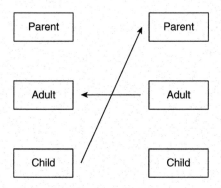

Figure 3.5 A crossed transaction

Non-verbal communication and transactional analysis

Transactional analysis is not just about what people say. It includes body language, attitudes and other non-verbal cues such as tone of voice. Cork and Ferns (2008) give examples of each state, illustrating typical phrases, behaviour and attitudes, as shown in Table 3.1.

Table 3.1 Summary of the transactional model

Ego state	Typical words and phrases	Typical behaviour	Typical attitudes
Critical parent	Disgraceful, ought, should, always	Furrowed brow, pointing, hands on hips	Condescending, judgemental
Nurturing parent	Well done, there there	Benevolent smile, pat on back	Caring, permissive, reassuring
Adult	How? When? Where?	Relaxed, attentive	Open minded, inquiring, interested
Adapted child	Please can I?, I'll try harder	Vigorous head nodding, whiny voice	Compliant, defiant, complaining
Natural child	I want, I feel great!, Wow!	Uninhibited, laughing	Curious, fun-loving, spontaneous

Source: Cork and Ferns, 2008

Positions

Harris (1973) summarised the states people tend to adopt as being 'OK' or 'not OK'. Someone who has a positive self-concept, shaped by positive strokes from others from childhood, will be OK and will treat others as OK. In other words, they will take a positive responsibility for themselves and expect others to be able to do the same. This would result in adult–adult transactions.

However, a parent-to-child transaction would be 'I'm OK – you're not OK', because the 'parent' sees themselves as 'better' than the other.

Table 3.2 summarises the typical **positions** people can take, often habitually, in certain circumstances.

Table 3.2 Positions in transactional analysis

Position	Attitude
I'm OK – you're OK	I am confident, capable and have self-worth, and I presume you do too.
I'm OK – you're not OK	I am capable and powerful but you are in need (positive).
I'm OK – you're not OK	I am capable and powerful but you are weak and worthless (negative).
I'm not OK – you're OK	I can't cope but you can and I need you.
I'm not OK – you're not OK	We are both (or all) worthless so there is no point in anything.

A good rule of thumb for the nurse delivering the principles of self-care and empowerment is that every nurse–patient transaction is from the 'I'm OK – you're OK' position.

There are times, though, when it is therapeutic to adopt a different position. In the crossed transaction example above, we saw a patient in the 'I'm not OK – you're OK' position and needing reassurance in an 'I'm OK – you're not OK' position from the doctor. In health promotion, it is important to make patients aware when they would benefit from changing their behaviour. Take alcohol misuse, for example. A patient with alcohol-related liver disease will need to stop drinking to maximise their recovery, or even to prevent death. It is very common for people addicted to alcohol to be in denial and make statements like:

It won't happen to me.

I'd rather die young and happy than old and miserable.

I can't stop drinking – it's no good trying.

The first two statements are 'I'm OK', and the third is 'I'm not OK'.

To encourage someone to become aware of their problems we might want to change their 'I'm OK' position to 'I'm not OK'. However, we don't want them to become hopeless and fall into the fifth position of 'I'm not OK – you're not OK'.

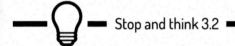

Stop and think 3.2

Can you think of any type of nursing circumstances where you would use the OK/not OK approach to communication in health promotion?

Suggested answer: did you think of things like encouraging smoking cessation, healthier eating and weight loss, compliance with medication regimes such as in self-care for diabetes or bipolar disorder, or in coming to terms with changed body image challenges following a stroke or acquired disability?

When someone needs to accept help, the ideal nurse–patient relationship would be 'I'm OK – you're not OK'. This way the nurse becomes a source of hope for the patient. Look at the exchange in Box 3.3.

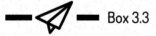

Box 3.3

Changing positions (1)

Patient: 'I like to drink. It's what makes life fun.'

Nurse: 'It's not fun when you get the shakes though, is it?'

(Continued)

Patient: 'No, but I just have another!'

Nurse: 'And how long do you think that can go on for?'

Patient: 'You're right, I know. But I don't like to think about it.'

The patient has moved on from 'I'm OK' statements to an 'I'm not OK – you're OK' position (note: 'you're right' and 'but I don't like … ' mean 'you can but I can't'). Look at the exchange in Box 3.4. The nurse adopts 'I'm OK – you're not OK' with this patient.

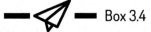 Box 3.4

Changing positions (2)

Nurse: 'I know it's hard for you right now. You can't see a way out.'

Patient: 'No, I can't. I don't see me being able to change.'

Nurse: 'I have heard many people like you say that. And they are now healthy and enjoying life.'

Patient: 'Really?'

The patient makes an 'I'm not OK' statement ('I can't change'), then responds to the nurse's 'I'm OK' position ('I know more than you') with recognition of the nurse's greater knowledge/power with 'really?'

This nurse–patient relationship has taken an 'I'm OK – you're not OK' position which provided some reality for the patient but also some hope that his situation can change through the help of others.

While it is usually problematic to encourage dependence on the nurse, in this case it is important that the patient engages with the treatment process in order to tackle the health problem. This use of communication skills and knowledge tends to apply to specialist care areas, which we will look at in later chapters.

Games and ulterior transactions

Very often, we use our 'positions' to manipulate others and get some kind of 'pay off'. Families are a rich source of **game-playing**, especially when there are teenagers around!

Everyone plays games, including in work teams, but most people do not know they're doing it and don't really intend to manipulate or hurt others.

A '**game**' is a series of habitual and unconscious interactions that attempt to manipulate other people. In other words, a game consists of a series of **ulterior transactions** where one position or ego state provides a subtle way of presenting another ego state. The clever put-down is a good example:

I see you still have that dress from last year. So lucky the fashion now is 'anything goes'.

This is an example of a nice adult ego state supposedly giving a positive stroke that actually delivers a critical parental message: 'you're out of fashion and I know better!' Game-playing involves a series of ulterior interactions that establish a fixed position for the player and manoeuvres others into co-responding positions.

Games can be played from any ego state but the aim of the transaction is to put others in a desired position. See Box 3.5.

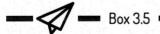 Box 3.5

Game-playing in a practice setting

The charge nurse of a day clinic called a meeting of all nursing staff at the end of the clinic. Everyone was waiting in the office for the meeting but the charge nurse was late. Two nurses (X and Y) popped next door to do some paperwork. The charge nurse appeared in the office and said 'where are nurses X and Y? Why are they late?' Someone fetched the two nurses and when they were in the office the charge nurse said to them (but really to everyone else in the room), 'try not to be late in future. You've kept all your colleagues waiting.'

Box 3.5 gives an example of very typical game-playing. The charge nurse felt guilty about being late and blamed the two missing nurses (scapegoating). The key is that it was done in front of the team so that the charge nurse could state 'I am not keeping you waiting – it's them'. The two nurses who were blamed will be aware of the charge nurse's real nature and feel aggrieved, but this may be lost on the rest of the team. The transaction puts the two nurses in the position of being at fault, while the charge nurse becomes the heroic defender of the other members of staff. This kind of game-playing is obviously bad for morale and teamwork, but in a team with an authoritarian leader (who assumes a critical parent ego state) it is all too common.

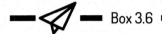 Box 3.6

Game–playing in patients' families

The mother of a young man with schizophrenia is very stressed by her carer role and is worried about how much longer she can care for her son. With the son present in the room, the mother tells the community psychiatric nurse that her son is becoming aggressive towards her and may do her some harm. He becomes annoyed at this accusation and forcefully denies this, saying he's fine but she winds him up. The mother then turns to the nurse and says, 'See, I can't say anything to him without him blowing up at me.'

Box 3.6 is an example of how patients and families may play games, with each other or with staff. The community nurse in this example could make the mistake of becoming part of the mother's game by agreeing with her. The nurse will gain the mother's trust in the short term, but lose the trust of the son. However, if the nurse is a good communicator, they will see the game as an expression of the mother's stress and recognise the threat to the son's stability due to this.

Games are not always destructive. Sometimes someone likes to be in the role of 'nurse' and constantly put themselves out to appear helpful and caring. Patients may appropriately put themselves in a dependent role when they are ill. We all play social games when we pretend to be interested in someone's story, appear pleased to be visiting the in-laws or look like we are enjoying someone's boring birthday party!

In nursing, it is important we develop our self-awareness in order to recognise when we are game-playing and when it is destructive to patients or colleagues. We also need to be aware of games even if they are not harmful. Games still stop us communicating realistically with others and allow others to play games.

Summary of transactional analysis

Transactional analysis is a very useful communication model because it helps the nurse to 'read' a person's emotional state and to respond appropriately. It is recommended as a useful framework for students to develop communication skills through training and **reflective practice** (Bailey and Baillie, 1996; Rowe, 1999). It is also shown to increase nurses' empathy and communication skills (Whitley-Hunter, 2014) and when nurses receive transactional analysis training it can improve patient satisfaction in their care and treatment (Sheikhmoonesi et al., 2013). The emphasis on developing an adult ego state in patients is seen as a useful tool in the promotion of **self-care** (Parissopoulos and

Kotzabassaki, 2004), and is identified as a tool to develop **clinical supervision** skills for supervisors and supervisees (Holyoake, 2000; McIntosh et al., 2006).

....

Knowledge link You will see how important supervision and reflective practice are to continuing professional development in Chapter 16.

....

Heron's six-category intervention analysis

John Heron (1975) devised a simple system for professional development training in interpersonal skills. This system allows the practitioner to look at their practice and identify what areas of communication they are good at and where they need to develop. He proposed that there are six main styles of intervention, all of which are used to deliver professional interpersonal communication. Health-related communication could be counselling, therapy, teaching, informing or interviewing, and may involve patients, relatives, colleagues or multi-disciplinary situations. Heron suggests that the different styles can be used for good when delivered with care and concern, but can be destructive when in a 'degenerate' form which serves the self-interest of the practitioner. This idea shows that communication skills are very powerful and need to be used with care when put into practice in the caring professions.

Table 3.3 lists Heron's six styles, or categories, of intervention, with examples of typical uses.

Table 3.3 Heron's six categories of intervention

Category	Uses
Authoritative *Prescriptive*: to give advice, be judgemental/critical/ evaluative. Seeks to direct the behaviour of the other.	i) Advising patient on medications on discharge ii) Demonstrating a procedure to a learner iii) Stopping a child scratching a rash
Informative: giving instruction, information, interpretation. Aims to give new knowledge to another.	i) Orienting a new patient to the ward ii) Presenting a patient at handover or to a multi-disciplinary team iii) Writing up nursing notes
Confronting: being challenging, giving direct feedback. Aims to challenge or question restrictive attitudes, beliefs or behaviour of others.	i) A mentor giving critical feedback on a student's timekeeping ii) A student questioning marks given for an assignment iii) A nurse telling a relative that aggressive behaviour is unacceptable
Facilitative *Cathartic*: release tension, encourage laughing, crying, expression of anger. Aims to enable others to get things off their chest ('abreaction' in Heron's description).	i) Providing a shoulder to cry on ii) Telling a joke in an embarrassing situation iii) Reassuring a child having a tantrum

(Continued)

Table 3.3 (Continued)

Category	Uses
Catalytic: facilitate problem-solving. Aims to enable self-learning in others.	i) Providing clinical supervision and reflective learning ii) Listening to someone talk through a problem iii) Providing play materials for children
Supportive: be approving, confirming, validating. Aims to show the other that they have worth and value.	i) All nursing situations ii) All teaching situations iii) All professional communications

The categories are divided into two main types: **authoritative** and **facilitative**. The authoritative styles of communication help the nurse adopt a power role to deliver healing in some form, where the patient does as the nurse indicates. This is the **paternalistic** approach in healthcare, or the 'doctor knows best' stance. It is appropriate in situations where the nurse needs to take the lead and adopt the more powerful position.

The facilitative styles help the patient find their own solutions and encourage self-care and self-healing. These styles are more in keeping with the patient-centred approach. The last facilitative style, **supportive**, is suggested to be the style that needs to be always present in any communication transaction, whether accompanied by, say, a **prescriptive** or **confronting** approach. For Heron, this is what makes the difference between effective beneficial communication and '**degenerate**' communication.

Heron (1975) states that health professionals have the greatest difficulty in practising the cathartic interventions; that is, encouraging people to express their emotions. This makes sense because we all find it difficult to deal with people who are crying or acting aggressively and we tend to steer clear of encouraging it for our own comfort. There will be occasions when you feel uncomfortable in certain nurse–patient situations, for example when breaking bad news or broaching a sensitive subject such as death, sexual health or abuse. We will look at such specific scenarios in later chapters, but this section outlines a key model for identifying and breaking down our communication skills to work on our strengths and weaknesses.

➕ **Knowledge link** Chapters 11 and 12 contain more information on breaking bad news and dealing with bereavement and loss.

In 1988, researchers Morrison and Burnard found that student nurses rated themselves most poor at cathartic and confronting styles of communication (Morrison and Burnard, 1989). But later Ashmore and Banks (1997) found that, after transactional analysis training, students felt good about managing emotional styles such as being supportive and cathartic, but less good at informing and confronting due

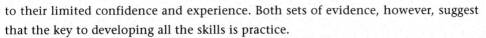

to their limited confidence and experience. Both sets of evidence, however, suggest that the key to developing all the skills is practice.

The skilful communicator, for Heron, is someone who:

• is proficient in all types of intervention
• can move easily between different styles as the situation requires
• is aware of what type of intervention they are using, and why.

Let's have a look at a real practice example by looking at the transcript in Practice example box 3.1 of a conversation between a female patient being admitted for a termination of pregnancy and a student nurse. The student has simply been instructed to carry out the admission procedure and is about to be landed with a bombshell. We come in during the orientation to the ward.

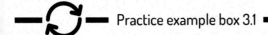 Practice example box 3.1

Transcript of a conversation

Nurse: 'This is your bed. You can put your things in the cabinet. If you have any valuables, I suggest you put them in the safe in the office.'

Patient: 'What shall I do with my bag? It's too big to fit in there.'

Nurse: 'Oh, how about putting it under the bed? That won't be in anyone's way. I'll leave you to get settled. I suggest you get changed into the gown as the anaesthetist will be doing his rounds soon.'

Patient: 'OK. Do I get to talk to someone, because I'm not sure I want to do this.'

Nurse: 'Oh, I see. Have you not gone over it with your doctor?'

Patient: 'Yes, but I'm not sure.'

Nurse: 'What are you not sure about? Is it the procedure itself or the termination?'

Patient: 'Well, I'm not worried about the op. I just ... I know everyone says it's the best thing to do but, I can't help feeling guilty. They say it's for my own good because I get really bad post-natal depression. And I have my other children to think of. But, what about this one too?'

Nurse: 'Yes, I see. You feel guilty about the termination but you'd feel guilty about your other children suffering when you get post-natal depression.'

(Continued)

Patient:	'Exactly. I can't win. I don't know what to do.' (looks distressed)
Nurse (sits beside the client on the bed and holds her hand):	'It's OK. You must feel very distressed. I can see you want to cry.'
Patient (starts crying):	'I don't know what to do.'
Nurse (puts arm round client):	'It's OK. I understand.'

This student nurse later questions the sister about this situation and finds out that the GP and the husband have persuaded her to have a termination. The patient is later offered counselling to help her make up her own mind.

The student nurse demonstrates all the styles of intervention during this episode. Her first approaches were authoritative and task-oriented – to inform and prescribe. She then had to adopt a **catalytic** style to help the patient explore what the problem was. When needed, she facilitated **catharsis** by being with the patient while she cried. Later, she used a confronting style to find out what was going on with this patient and question the manner in which she had agreed to the termination. This led to a more satisfactory approach for this patient to make her decision.

Can you spot which statements from the nurse indicate the style she is adopting? Be aware that they can overlap.

Summary of Heron's model

Heron's six-category intervention analysis is intended to be used to train and develop skills in communication for professionals. In nursing, reflective practice is an important part of the profession and we are obliged by the NMC *Code* (NMC, 2018) to maintain and enhance our skills. Heron's six-category intervention analysis can be used as a reflective practice tool for communication styles, and this is precisely what he designed it for. It has also been recommended for developing supervision skills by Sloan and Watson (2001). You can see more on using Heron's model for supervision and reflection in Chapter 16.

Skills development

Below are two exercises that enable to you to assess and reinforce your learning of the two models of communication.

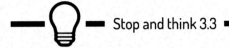

Stop and think 3.3

In Table 3.4 you will find a personal assessment sheet that can be used for skills assessment and reflection. Consider what categories you think you are particularly good at and which categories you are not so good at. Then make an action plan in order to seek opportunities in practice to develop these skills.

Table 3.4   Heron's six-category intervention analysis: personal assessment sheet

Identify the two categories that you feel you are *most* skilled in using at the present time, and the two categories that you feel you are *least* skilled in using at the present time

Category	Most skilled	Least skilled
Prescriptive		
Informative		
Confronting		
Cathartic		
Catalytic		
Supportive		

Now make an action plan to help you work on your skills

Skill assessment	I need to improve these elements of this skill ...	I will work on these skills by ...
Category 1 I am least skilled in ... because ...		
Category 2 I am least skilled in ... because ...		

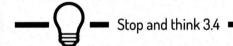

Stop and think 3.4

Now that you have identified your learning needs through self-assessment, below are some suggestions for you to develop your skills in transactional analysis and intervention analysis.

Choose a drama or soap opera on television that involves characters interacting verbally and non-verbally in typical social situations. Watch a dramatic scene where two people are interacting and take note of the styles of interaction each character adopts. Try to identify the ego states on display and note what it is about the words or behaviour that indicates which

(Continued)

ego state is being used. Why do you think that character is adopting that style? What does the other person do in response? Are the styles that are being used helpful or unhelpful to the situation? Why?

Obviously, the programme you choose is fictional, but the script writers and actors will portray dramatic communication behaviour. You may have found that a dramatic scene was not an adult–adult transaction! If you find this exercise easy, you are on the way to being able to 'read' others' communication styles and identify its effect on relationships.

You can also undertake Stop and think 3.4 by observing others in real life. Take some time out of a social situation or while on the ward to observe the interaction of others. You can identify what ego states people are adopting and also what happens when they change. Check with your mentor by relating your observations and see if they agree with you. This is also a skills development exercise in reflection and supervision.

Conclusion

The two models of communication we have looked at in this chapter have helped professionals structure their understanding of the skills and enabled assessment and development of skill deficits. Transactional analysis particularly aids the nurse in delivering client-/patient-centred care and to move away from a more traditional patriarchal style of healthcare that existed in the past. Heron's six-category intervention analysis helps the professional develop their skills in communicating, especially where a caring and concerned approach is required.

The first step to developing our communication skills is to identify what we already do, what we do well and what we do less well. Models help us to identify what we are doing and give us guidelines for developing other areas of our practice. Both these models are demonstrated to be useful for skills development in health and social care and enable the student and qualified nurse to improve their communication skills in all areas of their professional practice.

FURTHER READING

Berne, E. (1964) *Games People Play*. Harmondsworth, Penguin Books.

Burnard, P. (2005) *Counselling Skills for Health Professionals* (4th edn). Cheltenham, Nelson Thornes.

Harris. T. (1973) *I'm OK – You're OK*. London, Pan Books.

Heron, J. (2001) *Helping the Client: A Practical Guide* (5th edn). Thousand Oaks, CA, SAGE Publications.

Rogers, C. (1957) The necessary and sufficient conditions of therapeutic personality change. *Journal of Consulting Psychology*, 21, 95–103.

....REFERENCES

Ashmore, R. and Banks, D. (1997) Student perceptions of their interpersonal skills: a re-examination of Burnard and Morrison's findings. *International Journal of Nursing Studies*, 34(5), 335–345.

Bailey, J. and Baillie, L. (1996) Transactional analysis: how to improve communication skills. *Nursing Standard*, 10(35), 39–42.

Berne, E. (1964) *Games People Play*. Harmondsworth, Penguin Books.

Cork, A. and Ferns, T. (2008) Managing alcohol related aggression in the emergency department (part II). *International Emergency Nursing*, 16, 88–93.

Harris, T. (1973) *I'm OK – You're OK*. London, Pan Books.

Heron, J. (1975) *Six Category Intervention Analysis: The Human Potential Research Project*. Guildford, University of Surrey, Centre for Adult Education.

Holyoake, D. (2000) Using transactional analysis to understand the supervisory process. *Nursing Standard*, 14(33), 37–41.

McIntosh, N., Dircks, A., Fitzpatrick, J. and Shuman, C. (2006) Games in clinical genetic counselling supervision. *Journal of Genetic Counseling*, 15(4), 225–243.

Morrison, P. and Burnard, P. (1989) Students' and trained nurses' perceptions of their own interpersonal skills: a report and comparison. *Journal of Advanced Nursing*, 14, 321–329.

NMC (2018) *The Code: Professional Standards of Practice and Behaviour for Nurses, Midwives and Nursing Associates*. www.nmc.org.uk/standards/code/.

Parissopoulos, S. and Kotzabassaki, S. (2004) Orem's Self-Care Theory, transactional analysis and the management of elderly rehabilitation. *ICUs and Nursing Web Journal*, 17, 11.

Rowe, J. (1999) Self-awareness: improving nurse-client interactions. *Nursing Standard*, 14(8), 37–40.

Sheikhmoonesi, F., Zarghami, M., Tirgari, A. and Khalilian, A. (2013) Effect of transactional analysis education to nurses on patients' satisfaction. *European Psychiatry*, 28(S.1), Article 465. https://linkinghub.elsevier.com/retrieve/pii/S092493381375791 (accessed 25 June 2019).

Sloan, G. and Watson, H. (2001) John Heron's six-category intervention analysis: towards understanding interpersonal relations and progressing the delivery of clinical supervision for mental health nursing in the United Kingdom. *Journal of Advanced Nursing*, 36(2), 206–214.

Whitley-Hunter, B.L. (2014) Validity of transactional analysis and emotional intelligence in training nursing students. *Journal of Advances in Medical Education and Professionalism*, 2(4), 138–145.

FOUR

ACTIVE LISTENING AND ATTENDING: COMMUNICATION SKILLS AND THE HEALTHCARE ENVIRONMENT

EULA MILLER AND LUCY WEBB

THIS CHAPTER WILL HELP YOU TO:

- Take a person-centred approach to care
- Make appropriate use of the environment, self and skills
- Project warmth, sensitivity and compassion
- Listen, observe and respond to verbal and non-verbal cues
- Having insight into own values
- Use active listening, questioning, paraphrasing and reflection
- Empower people to meet their own needs and make choices

Introduction

In this chapter we will describe and demonstrate how basic communication skills are applied in practice. We will explain the techniques used in conducting an effective assessment or therapeutic conversation in healthcare settings, using guidelines, tips and practice examples to underline and demonstrate the techniques. The first half of the chapter will look at the basic skills underpinning communication skills that are part of the NMC's *Future Nurse: Standards of Proficiency for Registered Nurses* (NMC, 2018) for communication and managing relationships, and the second half will look at general frameworks that support effective interviews, consultations and patient assessments.

Core skills of effective communication

Whether we are conducting a formal interview or assessment, or taking the opportunity to converse with a patient to establish a good relationship, when we have any conversation, with anybody, there are some key basic skills that we can develop to improve our relationship-building, information-finding or information-giving. All these are essential to good nursing skills.

Active listening

Active listening is described as a form of communication that aids the nurse in listening attentively to the patient but also *shows* the patient they are being listened to (Wegner et al., 2014). Active listening encourages the patient to give information, express concerns and generally communicate what is important to them in their care. In turn, the nurse can then structure care around the patient's holistic needs. Active listening can be effective in overcoming cultural divides between the nurse and patient (Hart and Mareno, 2013; Crawford et al., 2017), improving the patient's sense of self-reliance, empowerment and, most importantly, feeling that their best interest is at the core of care given (Cope et al., 2016). Its absence can result in patients feeling abandoned psychologically, and not listened to (Sonis et al., 2016). Active listening is also recommended for multi-disciplinary interactions; for example, handovers in clinical areas (Burgener, 2017).

Active listening is an essential skill that is required by the NMC (2018) and supports the nurse–patient relationship (Conroy et al., 2017). In order to develop an effective nurse–patient relationship we need to employ essential communication skills in:

- attending
- hearing
- understanding
- remembering
- responding
- evaluating.

(Brownell, 2015)

To engage in active listening, the nurse also needs to enable it to take place. The skills above rely on the nurse being able to:

- create a conducive environment
- manage their time
- provide authentic (genuine) non-judgemental support and concern.

(Nelson-Jones, 2013)

Attending refers to the process of 'tuning in' or 'being there' – physically and psychologically. This process requires the health professional to use **active listening** skills. Active listening encompasses appropriate eye contact (which shows that you are interested in what is being communicated) and appropriate response to cues. This response needs to be balanced with not interrupting before the patient has completed important statements and hearing and detecting the meaning the patient's statements have for them. Active listening could be described as *hearing between the lines*.

Communication skills are often assessed in a practical examination called an Objective Structured Clinical Examination (OSCE). OSCEs are popular forms of assessment in healthcare education as they can measure competency in practical and clinical skills. You are likely to be required to demonstrate your active listening skills in practice in a communication skills OSCE. This will involve your reflection on key aspects of the listening skills you employ during a nurse–patient encounter, including how well you listened and heard what the patient said. We can often be distracted from attending to what the patient is saying because we are planning our next question! How well do you actually hear and understand what the patient is saying?

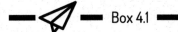 Box 4.1

Example of active listening

A young man who had been admitted for accidental overdose of heroin was being assessed by a nurse for drug use. While giving the history of his heroin use, the young man said he was experienced in drug injecting and did not have accidents. Because of the quietness of this statement, the lowered eyes and distracted fiddling with his sheets, this appeared to be a significant statement for this man to make. After sensitive exploring by the nurse, it was revealed that his overdose was actually an intentional suicide attempt and he still felt that he wanted to die. He stated later that no one during his admission had sat down with him and listened carefully enough for him to disclose this.

Box 4.1 illustrates the core skills of active listening. The nurse *listened* to and *heard* what the patient was saying and assessed the situation in order to *understand* what he meant. The nurse was able to *remember* the details already gained from the patient to put what was said into context. Importantly, the nurse had facilitated the active listening encounter with this patient by giving time and attention, providing the appropriate environment and gaining enough of his trust for him to confide this to someone. His statement was, to all intents and purposes, a plea for help.

Throughout this book, you will read more material on active listening that authors put into different practice contexts. Active listening is at the heart of professional communication and underpins all effective communication with patients, relatives and colleagues. It is especially important in taking an accurate history and gaining insight into the patient's needs for delivering holistic care. It underpins the nurse–patient relationship by establishing an empathetic relationship and conveying non-judgemental regard and interest from the nurse.

Asking questions

Active listening is supported by asking the right questions. We can guide the other person by turning the direction of the discussion through our questions. In this way, the nurse exercises a degree of power over the other person by setting and controlling the agenda. How we do this depends on what types of questions we ask. Firstly, we need to ensure the other person knows what we are asking.

Be clear

Questions to patients, relatives or fellow professionals need to be clear and understandable. A question to a child needs to be put in simpler terms than a question to a consultant surgeon, but both the child and the consultant need to understand what information we want from them. To be clear, it is usually easier to ask one question at a time. This sounds obvious until you try to ask a complex question that has conditions and contingencies. For example:

> 'If you were to go home today, and you had support from your daughter, would that be easier for you than if we set up a home help for you?'

Why not just ask:

> 'Would you prefer to go home today and be looked after by your daughter, or wait til we can arrange a home help?'

Using closed questions

Closed questions elicit 'yes', 'no' or other single-word answers. These are great if you have a patient who is very easily distracted such as a young child, an intoxicated or psychotic patient or someone with major learning difficulties. An easy way to elicit answers is to ask questions that can be answered with a single-word answer such as 'yes' or 'no', or forced-choice questions which give the person a single choice (Burnard, 2006):

'Do you want a cup of tea?' Yes/no

'How many sugars do you want in your tea?' Single-word answer

'Is the pain worse in your leg or your foot?' Forced-choice question

Using open questions

Open questioning can elicit more complex answers. They are much better at getting lots of information in an assessment or encouraging a patient to talk about a topic in more detail (Burnard, 2006). People are often reluctant to talk about illness or their personal situations, but a string of open questions can let the person know that you are interested in the answers and that the patient is making a great contribution to their care by answering them.

In an assessment or interview, open questions are often started with inquiring words such as *when, what, why, who, where* or *how*. This is often referred to as the **5WH** (see Box 4.2).

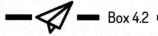 Box 4.2

The 5WH of open questioning

What: what happened when you went to your GP?

Why: why did you go to your GP?

Who: who supports you when you feel stressed?

Where: where do you think you get your anxiety from?

When: when do you feel like having a cigarette?

How: how does the asthma affect your child?

Exploring: sequential and circular questioning

Open questions help us to explore a topic with the service user, but sometimes the service user doesn't know the answers or, at least, has not really considered the issue in depth before. In this case, we need to adopt exploratory styles in our conversation.

We can adopt various styles of questioning which have been shown to be particularly effective for exploring issues, particularly in family or group situations (Kolbe et al., 2016). Two of these are called **sequential** and **circular questioning**.

Sequential questions aim to make visible patterns of behaviour, symptoms, effects, experiences and so on. They are often direct and follow a sequence of events. For example:

> 'How did you feel when you were told you had cancer? How do you feel now? How will you feel when you start treatment?'

Such questioning will make the person think about the topic specifically in relation to circumstances. The questions may help them come to terms with their feelings and anticipate the future. Another example may be:

> 'When did you first experience the pain? What were you doing at the time? What makes the pain worse now?'

This will give the nurse information about the symptoms and aid assessment and diagnosis.

Circular questions are even more exploratory. They assist in looking at the issue from a different viewpoint. Sometimes this can give new insight into a problem that the interviewee didn't have before. The questions aim to make the interviewee consider or imagine the issue from someone else's perspective, or their own perspective in a different time or place. For example:

- How do you think your husband views your behaviour when you are depressed?
- Before you were ill, how would you regard someone like you with your problems?
- What do you think most people would say about your behaviour?
- Why would they say that?

This type of questioning is very useful when dealing with groups or families (Kolbe et al., 2016; Holtslander et al., 2013). For example, in a family therapy session with parents of an anorexic teenager and the younger brother present, the interviewer could ask the younger brother:

> 'In your opinion, what does Jane do when she feels angry?'

As you will see in Chapter 5, the dynamics of groups are complex and very often people have fixed ways of thinking about themselves and others. By asking people to comment on others, people often let down their guard and say what they really feel. This affects not just them, but the other members of the group. Group work and family therapy is a specialised form of therapeutic communication, but all nurses can adopt some of the techniques of questioning to assess or explore specific problems.

Socratic questioning

Socratic questioning is a very useful technique for establishing a mutual relationship between the nurse and the interviewee, and helping the other to discover ideas for themselves. It uses a simple strategy of pursuing a line of questioning until all the details are revealed. What the interviewer is usually aiming for is the underlying reason a person behaves or thinks the way they do. This is as much for the interviewee to learn as for the interviewer's enlightenment.

See the following example:

Interviewer: 'Why do you not like attending the self-help group?'

Interviewee: 'I am not sure.'

Interviewer: 'Why do you feel unsure?'

Interviewee: 'Sometimes it feels crowded.'

Interviewer: 'What's wrong with it being crowded?'

Interviewee: 'There are too many people listening to me.'

Interviewer: 'What's wrong with being listened to?'

Interviewee: 'If I say something everyone will think I am stupid.'

Interviewer: 'Why do you think they will think you're stupid?'

Interviewee: 'Because I can't explain myself well.'

Interviewer: 'Is that because they won't understand what you mean?'

Interviewee: 'No, but my ideas make me feel ashamed.'

Interviewer: 'What do you feel ashamed of?'

Interviewee: 'I don't know. I guess that's the real problem, isn't it?'

Notice how the interviewer pursues the topic in detail. The interviewer might well have a good idea of where the problem lies, but needs the interviewee to explore it themselves. This way, the interviewee gets a sense of identifying their own problem.

Focusing

Questions can be either broad and exploring, or narrowed and specific. Both have important roles. Often, broad questioning about a topic helps in the beginning of an interview, before we switch to more specific questions for more detailed information. Broad questions are often very open, and focused questions can become almost closed questions.

Let's say we want to know how the behaviour of a patient with dementia is affecting the informal carer. We may ask at first:

'What sort of behaviours do you find most difficult to cope with?'

We find out that the main problem is wandering, so focus on that aspect of the patient's safety management by using a closed question:

'What would happen if you put locks on all the external doors? Would you feel guilty about keeping him in?'

In this example, the questioning goes from broad to focused.

Attending

Active listening and attending rely on being able to communicate to the other person that we *are* listening, understanding, remembering and interested in what they are communicating. We need to focus on what we and the patient are communicating in order to create a sense of 'mutuality' in the conversation. Mutuality will be addressed later in this chapter but, for now, let's focus on the basics. There are some simple rules and tips to adhere to in order to get the basics right.

We can 'listen' to our patients in three key ways:

1   Verbally   what is said (or not said)
2   Vocally   how it is verbalised
3   Non-verbally   what body language is displayed

We can also influence all of these by the questions we ask, the way we ask and respond to them, and the body language we use when talking and listening.

Verbal attending: paraphrasing

One really good way to show the person we are listening is to use **paraphrasing**. This is simply repeating back to the person what you understand by what they've said, usually in your own words. This tells them that you are listening and understand them and helps you check that you have understood what they are trying to say:

'So, you're saying you don't like this medication because of the side effects?'

Vocal attending

Vocal attending involves the vocal noises and responses we make and the way we use our voice, rather than just what we say. Such as:

Grunts – 'ah–ha', 'yep', 'tut–tut'

Reflective responses – 'I see', 'I know what you mean', 'No, really?'

Tone, style and pace of voice – loud, excitable, fast paced, agitated, angry or slow, deliberate, quiet, thoughtful, distracted.

Non-verbal attending

Non-verbal attending can include body language, positioning/proximity, eye contact and general appearance. Also, it relates to both the nurse and the other person involved in communicating. We will look at non-verbal attending in the section on body language.

Body language

Body language refers to the gestures, physical attitude, behaviour and eye contact we adopt when conversing. We can use these to convey different messages to our patients but need to be aware what we are conveying as it is easy to give one message verbally and another message accidentally through our body language. For instance, I tend to get very tired at the end of a long day but am very aware I must not yawn too much when conducting an evening interview!

We can convey interest and concern by leaning forward slightly, using an open posture (not crossing our arms or legs) and using hand gestures and facial expressions to match the emotional message, such as surprise, shock, worry, support and joy. An underrated form of body language is *smiling*! If we give our patients a genuine smile they may not smile back but our warmth will register and make some small change in the contact between us and the patient.

We can also 'read' the other person by their body language. Defensive postures such as folded arms, facing away or poor eye contact tell us that the other person is feeling anxious or threatened in some way. Often, the body language accompanying what is being said can speak volumes about the importance of a statement.

Proxemics and messages of appearance

Proxemics refers to 'personal space', or the proximity of people to each other and the body zones that are acceptable for touching – or viewing. Both vary greatly between cultures and the type of relationship between people. Hugman (2009) suggests that people have a psychological spatial safety zone around them and infringement of that zone makes them feel uncomfortable. The zone may vary from person to person, influenced by personality and culture. However, it is important that two people sharing a space 'read' and respond to the other person's signals that signify the boundary of their comfort zone. How much a person is seen as a threat or a welcome contact depends on how they regard the other person. For instance, a 'motherly' stranger may be seen as less threatening and given more access than a stranger who comes across as authoritarian. Someone who reminds us of someone close and loved will not be as likely to 'violate' our space as someone who reminds us of a disliked figure. Behaviour that can violate personal space can be closeness, or proximity, touching and even eye contact. Looking at someone too intensely can be an intrusion of their comfort zone.

Nurses delivering hands-on care frequently have to encroach upon someone's spatial comfort zone. It is important that nurses recognise how the other person is reacting to our physical presence and approach. This is particularly important with people who cannot move away or communicate their anxiety or discomfort, for example a person with a brain injury or people with severe learning difficulties. See the example in Box 4.3.

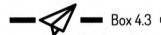 **Box 4.3**

Awareness of proxemics

An older man in a nursing home needed anti-Parkinsonian medication very early in the morning, often while he was still asleep. He had been in a Japanese prisoner of war camp where he experienced very cruel treatment. This man had frequent flashbacks of his time in the prison camp when waking, often panicking when people were too close to him. The nurse waking him to give the medication needed to approach very slowly and make it clear that she was a nurse and that he was safe in bed so that he wouldn't be alarmed and try to get away.

Any message that we can use to communicate 'safety' or 'non-threatening' to help patients feel comfortable with nursing intimacy is worth considering. For example, a disoriented older patient is likely to feel threatened when being bathed by a stranger, unless the stranger is clearly in a nurse's uniform and behaving as the older patient would expect a nurse to behave. Very often, the nurse's uniform gives a reassuring message to patients that it's OK to let us bathe them, toilet them, discuss intimate details with them and hold their hand when they are upset or frightened. For some, however, the uniform can be authoritarian and intimidating. With each patient we need to consider carefully how we come across in appearance. There are many factors to consider and some will be particular to individual patients. However, there are some general factors worth thinking about. Firstly, we could consider our sex, age and general appearance (i.e. tall, bearded, petite, youthful, mature and experienced). For instance, I know sometimes I come across as a bit scary – super-efficient but brusque and matter of fact – and have found that timid patients will often feel more at ease initially with my more 'mumsy' colleagues. This is something that nurses tend to gain insight into as they get practice experience and feedback from patients and colleagues. Learn what your limitations are because it will help you understand how and what you are communicating.

Eye contact and line of sight

Eye contact is a form of body language, but a very important one. It is a very primitive form of communication and contact with others. It is a peculiarity to humans that we have the whites of our eyes showing, unlike all other mammals. It is suggested by Mark Elgar (Aeria, 2016) that this makes humans much more sensitive to 'reading' other people – we can see where they are looking! Just think how you might feel when talking to someone wearing sunglasses compared to someone without sunglasses, or talking to someone who looks away from you all the time. Uncomfortable! Eye contact usually comes naturally to people who are normally sociable and not anxious. Often, people with autism find it very anxiety-provoking to look someone in the eye or to be looked at. When we are anxious or distracted, however, our eye contact can send a message that we would prefer not to engage or are wary. For example, a nurse who is concerned for their own safety with an angry patient can express anxiety through evasive eye contact or staring. A nurse who is anxious about the time will look at their watch. The patient will easily pick up on our true state of interest or arousal by our eye contact. Likewise, we can assess the state and even honesty of our patient by noting their eye contact.

Eye contact and line of sight can represent the balance of power between two people. Imagine two people conversing: one is in a wheelchair and one is crouching down to have a level eye line contact. How much more difficult would it be for the person in the wheelchair to converse if the other person was standing up? What if the other person was pushing the wheelchair from behind? Maintaining an equal eye line is often challenging in nursing where a patient may be in bed or sitting while the nurse is standing. Some little thought, and often a simple action, can go a long way to help the patient feel empowered. How easy is it to sit or squat by the patient to gain an equal line of sight?

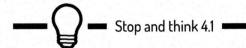 Stop and think 4.1

Next time you are in a public place with people around sitting or standing in conversations with each other, note how two people use their body language to convey meaning to the other. Even if you can't hear what they're saying, see if you can guess what they are talking about. Most importantly, when you've made a guess, identify what it was about their body language that gave you that impression.

Communicating for the assessment of needs

In a consultation or assessment interview we have a formal conversation with a patient or relative in order to assess their care needs. The nurse needs to structure the conversation to gain specific information. Sometimes this is already stipulated in an assessment form. However, the nurse should also gather more personal information from the patient or relative which will help to personalise care. Where the information needed is likely to be highly personal or individual, for example assessing a patient's stress, the assessment will need to be quite flexible and the nurse will need to 'think on their feet'. We will call this formal conversation an interview, although different specialties and fields of care have a range of terminology for a formal assessment of needs.

Before you begin

Have a clear goal in mind for a formal assessment. What do you want to know? How are you going to approach the patient and what barriers are likely to be in place?

Think about the setting. Where will this interview take place? Can you cut out communication barriers, for example noise, interruptions, distraction and discomfort? Ensure that you and your patient are dressed appropriately to put the patient at ease, and choose a time that is convenient to both parties. Arrange furniture, lighting and other environmental factors for comfort and ease for both of you (see Box 4.4). Be aware of who else might be in the room and within earshot, be it another professional, a relative or other patients. Ensure you have everything you need for the interview beforehand such as pen and paper, any assessment forms, information sheets for the patient or notes.

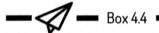 Box 4.4

The importance of environment

A sexual health nurse was asked to see a patient with a sexually transmitted disease on a general medical ward. The purpose of the interview was to take a history with the aim of referring the patient to the genitourinary medicine clinic.

The patient was in an eight-bedded bay on a very busy medical ward. On arrival and following initial introductions, it was clear that there would be no privacy at the bedside to elicit the patient's history. The nurse found the only empty space on the ward – the linen cupboard! The interview was conducted there very successfully. The unusual setting helped the patient feel his needs were being taken seriously and this built a good working relationship with the nurse from then on.

Starting the interview

Start by putting the patient at ease as soon as possible. Introduce yourself in a mutually respectful way and ensure the patient is immediately aware that you respect them as an equal but that this is a professional interview (see setting boundaries, Chapter 2).

The first sentences should be introductory, and reveal your human side. Seek to get the patient to relax and talk to you and don't be dominating. Set down the rules for the meeting with the patient – you must have their agreement (consent!), co-operation and achieve mutual respect. You need to inform the patient:

- how long the interview is likely to take
- the purpose of the interview
- what is to be discussed.

Ending the interview

Finishing an interview well is as important as starting. If you have told the patient or relative when you will finish, you need to keep to that agreement, or check that it is OK if you finish at a different time. It is important to keep the patient informed of how the interview is progressing. The person will feel a little more in control of the process and also know when they will get the opportunity to disclose important information or ask questions. Throughout the interview, tell the person how the process is going and how much further there is to go! Near the end, it is helpful to 'telegraph' the ending in some way. This helps the patient anticipate the end. It is surprising how often people will disclose something important at the last minute as they know it will be their last chance! To telegraph the end, the nurse can use phrases such as:

- 'I only have a couple of questions left.'
- 'We will have to finish in about 5 minutes.'
- 'I must leave you soon as your lunch will be here any minute.'

....

Knowledge link See Chapter 7 for more information on how to structure an interview or consultation.

....

Emotional intelligence and the therapeutic use of self

Therapeutic relationships form the foundation of all nursing work.

The therapeutic use of self is where the nurse uses personal strengths, experiences, understanding of human behaviour and communication skills to interact purposefully with the patient (Videbeck, 2009). This process, and the insight it affords, is collectively known as emotional intelligence and focuses on the nurse's understanding of self, i.e. how one's behaviour, attitudes and attributes have the potential for impact on others within the working environment. Nurses need emotional intelligence to practice effectively and to enhance their therapeutic interactions with recipients of care, family members, the public and all those individuals within the organisations in which they work (Fitzpatrick, 2016).

Therapeutic use of self in nursing is a phrase adapted from counselling which describes how the nurse can facilitate some form of healthy change in the patient through the nurse–patient relationship. The therapeutic use of self, and the building of this therapeutic alliance, is essential because it directly focuses on the needs, feelings, experiences and ideas of the patient only. We will look at some key examples below but first we need to look at how the nurse ensures that their relationship and communications with patients generally benefit the patient's health rather than detract from it.

Knowledge link This section adds to the introduction to the nurse–patient relationship covered in Chapter 2. Look back and remind yourself of the basic elements of the nurse–patient relationship.

Self-awareness

Key to the effective delivery of care through communication skills is the nurse's self-understanding and the use of self to communicate ideas to others. This is essential in marking the amount of sharing in the nurse–patient encounter and aids the depth of the material addressed by the nurse and patient. Chapter 2 introduced the notion of the nurse–patient relationship and the importance of self-awareness on the part of the nurse. In order to understand the patient, the nurse needs to understand how the patient is receiving the communication from the nurse. That requires the nurse to have good self-awareness about how they present to others and what messages they may consciously and unconsciously be giving out. See Box 4.5 for a simple example of where this might be important.

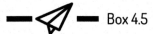 Box 4.5

The importance of appearance

A nurse dressed in surgical theatre scrubs approaches a 90-year-old woman on a surgical ward. The nurse asks her if she would like tea or coffee. The patient replies that she doesn't want either as she has a train to catch. The nurse then asks the woman if she would like to go to the toilet. The woman replies, annoyed, that she has a cheek asking such personal questions and that she is a very silly girl because, obviously, if she went to the toilet now, she might miss her train. The woman dismisses the nurse in an abrupt manner with a wave of her hand.

The nurse presumes this woman is senile and is disoriented to time and place. It does not occur to the nurse that the uniform she wears bears no resemblance to a nurse's uniform, but rather she appears to be someone in overalls. The manner of her dress simply adds disorientation to the woman's confused state.

By understanding how we are seen, both physically and psychologically, we can understand the responses people make to us, and then anticipate how we should present ourselves to enhance good relating. In the above scenario, the nurse could have introduced herself to the woman and helped to orientate her to the hospital environment first before asking her questions.

Empathy and self-disclosure

To develop a good nurse–patient relationship, even in a short interaction, it helps to 'get on the right wavelength' as quickly as possible and show the patient that you are 'with' them. This is often referred to as **mutuality** (Cox, 1978). The nurse needs to be able to relate to all sorts of patients and have at least some understanding of their point of view. This does not mean agreement, but does allow the nurse to relate to the other's experience. The nurse also needs to show the patient that they have empathy, and this can be where a degree of self-disclosure is useful.

Self-disclosure is a tricky technique to use as it can overstep the mutuality boundary in the nurse–patient relationship. However, it can be useful to show a patient that you have experienced something similar or you can check if your experiences give you better insight into the patient. For example, a patient expressing fear of an operation may be reassured by a student nurse who discloses that they were also afraid of operations, until they saw what happens and realised that it was OK. A trickier disclosure might be when a patient expresses annoyance at a particularly brusque doctor and the nurse replies that, actually, everyone has trouble with his manner!

Self-disclosure can be useful, but must be carefully applied. It would be easy for the patient to assume we are, in effect, saying 'I know how you feel', when we only know how we felt in similar circumstances. Or we could be taking away the personal uniqueness of the patient's experience by giving the message, 'I had that too and I didn't make a fuss'. We need to be aware (self-aware) of why we are using self-disclosure and what kind of message the patient will receive from it. Is it to gain sympathy from the patient, or are we aiding the patient to recognise our empathy and therefore trust us a bit more? Are we using it solely to benefit the patient? Cox's work with mutuality and disclosure are well detailed in Burnard (2006).

Informing

Communication is used heavily for assessment and therapeutic engagement, as seen above. It is also, and particularly routinely, used to give information to patients, relatives and other service users, and to pass on relevant information to our colleagues. Chapters 12–15 will look at information-giving in greater detail, but we can be aware here that how we give information to others needs to be adapted so that the other person can understand the information. When giving information to other health professionals, we tend to give it in a formalised manner, using certain phrases and adopting medical-style language. We know what we are saying will be understood. When informing lay people (people not medically trained) we need to use active listening skills to assess how to give the information and whether it has been understood.

Matching information styles

Let's say our patient is a plumber. He is due to have a hernia operation. In order to give information, we could first explore what he already knows, and, crucially, how he understands it:

Interviewer:	'Tell me what you know about your problem.'
Interviewee:	'Well, I have a burst wall in my gut which is causing part of my insides to seep out.'
Interviewer:	'OK, do you know why it has to be fixed and how?'
Interviewee:	'I think so. It could get trapped, the doctor said, and cause that bit of gut to die. He said he has to stuff it back in and sew it up again to seal the hole.'

So, the interviewer has gained a good idea of both what the patient knows, and how he knows it. For good communication, the interviewer needs to put it into the patient's own terminology. Here, the practitioner knows how to explain any further procedures and recovery in similar terms.

Styles and levels of understanding become particularly important when dealing with children or people with cognitive difficulties. It is important to assess their understanding first or we could make assumptions about their inability to understand – and so patronise them – or assume too much ability and give them information which goes over their heads. With young children or people with cognitive difficulties, it is often useful to use pictures, diagrams or even play- or role-modelling to give information. Pictures are useful because they work at a concrete level of understanding. Concrete thinking helps us understand something particularly complex. It is easier to set it out on paper, in diagrams, or to use metaphors and similes. For example, I don't understand quantum physics and black holes, but I can picture a black hole in my mind as a giant whirlpool that sucks everything in!

Knowledge link See Chapters 5, 11 and 12 for communication with colleagues.

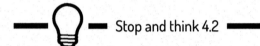

Stop and think 4.2

Have you ever noticed that doctors often refer to the abdomen as the 'tummy' when talking to patients? Why do you think this is? Do you think it's patronising?

Possible answer: doctors are trained to give information at the patient's level of understanding. In the past, doctors were renowned for speaking in medical language when talking to patients, who then needed the nurse to explain when the doctor had gone! However, they don't have time to assess the patient's own style or level of understanding so the best approach is for them to use simplified language with patients all the time. This has become stylised to some degree, so that certain medical words are converted into specific lay language, such as abdomen = tummy.

Motivating

Motivational communication is very important when we need to change someone's health behaviour or attitude to their health status. For instance, if someone is obese and at risk of type 2 diabetes, a nurse's health promotion role would be to encourage them to eat healthily and take exercise. Also, if someone develops an illness that needs self-care, the person may need encouragement to regard coping with the illness as a challenge rather than the end of their quality of life. Good skills in motivating are like clever advertising: they aim to persuade someone to change something about themselves – eat more salad or buy brand X soap powder! Motivational interviewing is an important and effective communication strategy in nursing, particularly in health promotion and for changing unhealthy behaviour (Naidoo and Wills, 2016).

The secret of active listening in motivational communication is, like informing, understanding how the person already regards the issue and their capability or desire to change. In short, we need to assess the person for changeable points. See Table 4.1 for verbal examples of a changeable point.

Table 4.1 Motivational changeable points

Changeable points	Verbal example
Current health beliefs	Once you've got cancer, that's it.
Current view of ability to change	I'm too fat to take exercise.
Current desire (motivation) to change	But I need a cigarette when I'm stressed.
Barriers that the person perceives	I'd eat salads more often if it wasn't for the kids. They like their chips!
Key factors to motivate them to change	I worry about how the family would cope if I wasn't here anymore.

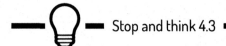 Stop and think 4.3

Look at the patient statements in Table 4.1. See if you can construct questions from the examples in this chapter that challenge those statements. Remember that you can use Socratic, circular, sequential, open or closed questions.

Suggested question styles:

- 'Once you've got cancer, that's it.' Do you think everyone thinks that? (circular questioning)
- 'I'm too fat to take exercise.' What about people who lose weight by exercising? Weren't they fat when they started? (closed, one-word answer)
- 'But I need a cigarette when I'm stressed.' What do you mean by 'need'? (Socratic questioning: pursue until the person defines need and realises they won't die if they don't have a cigarette.)
- 'I would eat salads more often if it wasn't for the kids. They like their chips.' What would happen if you had a salad and they had chips? (Sequential questioning aimed at challenging the assumption that this is unchangeable.)
- 'I worry about how the family would cope if I wasn't here anymore.' What could you do to ensure you were here for them? (A type of circular question that elicits an action statement: a step towards making a plan and taking action.)

As you can see, a patient's statements tell us what stops them adopting more healthy behaviour, and what might motivate them to change. In order to elicit these statements, we need to engage in active listening, questioning and attending.

Knowledge link See Chapters 9, 12 and 15 for more theory and practice in motivational communication.

Conclusion

Active listening and attending underpin all communication as they help the practitioner understand the patient's perspective and therefore what their communication needs are, and how to respond. It is called *active* listening because it describes what the practitioner needs to do (act) in order to *listen*. This chapter has focused on the basic verbal and non-verbal skills which allow us to 'read' the other person and also 'tell' the other person something about ourselves – by the way we act, move and present ourselves. Basic active listening and attending skills are essential to developing the nurse–patient relationship but also to delivering interventions such as assessment, information-giving and motivating. Further chapters will build on these skills in specific healthcare practice areas and for specific needs.

FURTHER READING

Burnard, P. (2006) *Counselling Skills for Health Professionals* (4th edn). Cheltenham, Nelson Thornes.

REFERENCES

Aeria, G. (2016) Why we show the whites of our eyes. *Go Figure.* https://pursuit.unimelb. edu.au/articles/why-we-show-the-whites-of-our-eyes.

Brownell, J. (2015) *Listening: Attitudes, Principles, and Skills* (subscription; University of Melbourne research report website). New York, Routledge.

Burgener, A.M. (2017) Enhancing communication to improve patient safety and to increase patient satisfaction. *The Health Care Manager*, 36(3), 238–243.

Burnard, P. (2006) *Counselling Skills for Health Professionals* (4th edn). Cheltenham, Nelson Thornes.

Conroy, T., Feo, R., Boucaut, R., Alderman, J. and Kitson, A. (2017) Role of effective nurse-patient relationships in enhancing patient safety. *Nursing Standard*, 31(49), 53–63.

Cope, V.C., Jones, B. and Hendricks, J. (2016) Residential aged care nurses: portraits of resilience. *Contemporary Nurse*, 52(6), 736–752.

Cox, M. (1978) *Structuring the Therapeutic Process*. London, Jessica Kingsley.

Crawford, T., Candlin, S. and Roger, P. (2017) New perspectives on understanding cultural diversity in nurse–patient communication. *Collegian*, 24(1), 63–69.

Fitzpatrick, J.J. (2016) Helping nursing students develop and expand their emotional intelligence. *Nursing Education Perspectives*, 37(3), 124.

Hart, P.L. and Mareno, N. (2014) Cultural challenges and barriers through the voices of nurses. *Journal of Clinical Nursing*, 23(15–16), 2223–2233.

Holtslander, L., Solar, J. and Smith, N.R. (2013) The 15-Minute Family Interview as a learning strategy for senior undergraduate nursing students. *Journal of Family Nursing*, 19(2), 230–248.

Hugman, B. (2009) *Healthcare Communication*. London, Pharmaceutical Press.

Kolbe, M., Marty, A., Seelandt, J. and Grande, B. (2016) How to debrief teamwork interactions: using circular questions to explore and change team interaction patterns. *Advances in Simulation*, 1(1), 29.

Naidoo, J. and Wills, J. (2016) *Foundations for Health Promotion* (4th edn). Oxford, Elsevier.

Nelson-Jones, R. (2013) *Introduction to Counselling Skills Texts and Activities* (4th edn). London, SAGE Publications.

NMC (2018) *Future Nurse: Standards of Proficiency for Registered Nurses*. www.nmc.org.uk/globalassets/sitedocuments/education-standards/future-nurse-proficiencies.pdf.

Sonis, J., Mort, E., Natsui, S., Goldsmith, A., Joseph, T., White, B., Raja, A. and Aaronson, E. (2016) Listening to our patients' concerns: a call to focus experience efforts on communication and compassion. *Annals of Emergency Medicine*, 68(4), S8.

Videbeck, S.L. (2009) *Mental Health Nursing* (1st edn; adapted for the UK by K. Ascott). London, Wolters Kluwer/Lippincott Williams & Wilkins.

Weger, J.H., Castle Bell, G., Minei, E.M. and Robinson, M.C. (2014) The relative effectiveness of active listening in initial interactions. *International Journal of Listening*, 28(1), 13–31.

FIVE
GROUPS AND TEAMWORK
LUCY WEBB

.... THIS CHAPTER WILL HELP YOU TO:

- Act appropriately in sharing information with others
- Work collaboratively with a multi-professional team and other agencies
- Challenge your own practice and that of others across the multi-professional team
- Take an effective role within the team, adopting the leadership role when appropriate

Introduction

Understanding how groups work and being able to work with others are vital skills in nursing. You have perhaps already experienced working with nursing and other healthcare students to explore and share knowledge together in teams. It is important that nurses learn the skills of teamwork because it is a key feature of the nurse's clinical role.

The Code: Professional Standards of Practice and Behaviour for Nurses, Midwives and Nursing Associates (NMC, 2018) stipulates that nurses must use effective communication to share information with colleagues and preserve the safety of those receiving care. In practice, we are expected to work co-operatively, share our skills and experience and at the same time respect the skill and experience of others and take advice when appropriate. We often share care management with other professionals from health and social care services and therefore need to use sophisticated communication and interpersonal skills to be effective team members. For many patient needs, the multi-disciplinary team is likely to include the medical team, ward or community-based nurses and key worker, social worker and specialist members such as dietitian, occupational therapist, psychologist or physiotherapist. Extended collaboration may include inter-agency working with professionals from education, the police or specialist voluntary sector workers. The principle of holistic and person-centred care means that care is delivered as an integrated package, recognising that aspects of health, social functioning and environmental factors all impact on the person's wellbeing. Therefore, multi-disciplinary team and inter-agency teamwork is vital in delivering holistic care.

As a student, you will be studying and learning in groups and be expected, as a team of students, to engage in self-directed study. This is often a challenge to students because the effect of being in a task-oriented group in itself is part of the learning journey: you will develop your self-awareness from the feedback from other group members and will develop the communication and interpersonal skills necessary to make a team function effectively.

This chapter will examine what teams are, what teamwork is and how teams work. The chapter will also identify what the implications are for communication skills development in both practice and academic roles for the student nurse.

Groups and group behaviour

There is a large body of evidence relating to groups and how they operate. Many of the principles for groups apply to workplace teams so we will look at the theories that help explain groups and group factors. There are different kinds of groups but we will focus on two of the most relevant to nursing: work groups (teams) and families.

People in groups do things that they wouldn't necessarily do as individuals. Somehow, being with others and sharing a 'group identity' changes individuals' behaviour and even how they see themselves.

Conformity and identity

People in groups tend to form a **social identity**. Psychological studies including famous experiments by Tajfel and Turner (1979) and Sherif et al. (1961) show how belonging to a group creates a common group identity and can create rivalry and divisions between groups (Box 5.1).

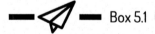 ▬ Box 5.1 ▬

Sherif et al.'s (1961) group identity studies

In a USA summer camp, researchers randomly assigned boys into two groups and encouraged them to socialise within their groups. After a week they brought the two groups together for a series of inter-group competitions. In the first week, the groups developed leaders and group norms and gave their groups names (Eagles and Red Devils). During the competition week, hostility broke out between the groups, even when not actively competing in activities such as watching TV or eating meals.

This type of evidence suggests we identify with the group we belong to and conform to the values and norms of that group, and identify who is not in our group: the out-group. This evidence, however, is based on artificial, experimental research with young people who, perhaps, do not have a well-developed sense of individual identity. But it can show how a lack of self-awareness can lead people into conforming behaviour.

Another well-known study of conformity is by Asch (1955) outlined in Box 5.2.

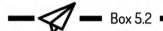 Box 5.2

Asch's (1955) study of conformity

A group of people were asked to match a line printed on a card with another line of equal length on another card. There was actually only one research subject in each group while all the others in the group were 'stooges' of the researchers. The lone subject did not know this. During the study procedure, the stooges constantly judged that the line matched another line of unequal length. This put pressure on the real subject to conform to the others' judgements, even though they may have thought their judgement wrong. Only around a quarter of the subjects actually disagreed with the other members of the group. Some even stated they believed the answer the others gave, so demonstrating conformity not just of behaviour but also of belief.

Evidence like this shows how the drive to conform to the group can be very strong, even to the point of changing the individual's own experience and creating doubt in their own perception. Such psychological theories of conformity and identity are often used to explain why people engage in destructive mob behaviour or join in with bullying. It is even thought to be fundamental to explaining the compliance with Nazi death camps and similar atrocities.

In a nursing context, a nurse may feel the pressure from the multi-disciplinary or nursing team to adopt an attitude or behaviour that they might not otherwise agree with as an individual. This conformity is not just about knowingly going along with others but actually adopting the same values as the others in the group. See Box 5.3 for a typical example.

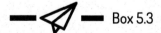 Box 5.3

Pressure to conform

A multi-disciplinary team was discussing the care plan for an older woman who lived alone and presented a risk to herself due to forgetfulness and disorientation. The key worker, an

(Continued)

inexperienced staff nurse, came to the meeting intending to recommend that the patient would have more support in her own home as a care home would increase the woman's disorientation and make her condition markedly worse. However, the other members of the team (consultant, social worker and charge nurse) all agreed that a care home placement was best. The staff nurse realised no one was going to agree with her. When asked her opinion, she agreed with the care home option. Although not comfortable with this idea, she thought that the others must know better and she was too inexperienced to recognise the dangers to this woman.

The staff nurse in the practice example in Box 5.3 appears to be socially inhibited by the pressure from the rest of the group, especially since they are more powerful and the nurse doesn't want to look inexperienced in front of the consultant and the charge nurse. The nurse in this situation changes perception of the risk this woman presents and supports the move to the care home.

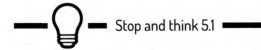 **Stop and think 5.1**

What difference would it make if the nurse in Box 5.3 had well-developed self-awareness? What role would assertiveness play in this situation?

Possible answer: nurses are often members of multi-disciplinary teams but may feel that issues relating more to nursing or the patient's needs are not valued compared to medical issues (Punshon et al., 2017). And yet it is often the nurse who knows the patient best and is in the best position to be an advocate for that patient (Punshon et al., 2017). A nurse in this situation would need to be aware of their own vulnerability to **conformity**, self-esteem needs (not to look naïve in front of other people) and feel confident enough to be assertive and dispute the group assumption that the woman should be in a care home.

Social roles

People in groups adopt different roles within the group, depending on what is needed and what suits the individual and other members of the group. This is often an unconscious process whereby people such as the leader will emerge. Often, someone may attempt to be the leader, but gradually the group will defer to someone else. A newly formed group will go through a process where these roles become clear. The roles adopted can be described as falling into two different categories: task roles and maintenance roles.

Task roles are those which focus on the task in hand – these are often the decision-maker, the problem-solver. The maintenance roles help the team work towards the task and keep the group together – these roles may be encourager, observer, peace-maker and leader. See Table 5.1 for a description of some of the common group roles identified by Benne and Sheats (1948) and Belbin (1981).

Table 5.1   Benne and Sheats' (1948) and Belbin's (1981) group roles

	Description
Benne and Sheats (1948) **Common roles of work groups**	
The encourager	Sees positive angles and provides good morale
The observer/commentator	Provides reflection on the group process; can be quiet
The joker	Diffuses difficulty; can be distracting
The recorder	Serves as the group's 'memory'
The agenda timekeeper	Helps the group stay on track
The critic	Sees the negative or problematic side
Belbin (1981) **Work 'types' and team participation**	
The 'plant'	Creative and good at solving problems
The coordinator	Confident; promotes joint decision-making
The team worker	Sociable, accommodating, listener
The completer-finisher	Conscientious, corrects errors
The specialist	Single-minded, dedicated

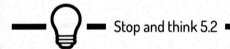 Stop and think 5.2

Consider a recent student group you have taken part in. This may have been as a small study group during a taught lecture or a problem-based learning group. What roles did people play? Was there a clear leader? Was there someone 'difficult' who caused problems? What was your role in the group? Observing group dynamics and your own role in groups will help develop your self-awareness in working with others.

In nurse education, small group work is widely used as it is valuable for learning complex material in depth and helps students develop collaborative skills (Jackson et al., 2014). However, work groups of this kind can be challenging. Often there are perceived problems of unequal workload sharing, poor leadership, disputes and blame. These are usually normal group dynamics that expose student nurses to the learning process of working and communicating in groups and teams. Let's look at typical group dynamics and processes.

Group dynamics

Any group of people who are forming a team will go through a process of group development towards some form of cohesion. Tuckman (1965) identified five developmental phases that can be seen in any type of group in which the group members adapt to roles, group identity is formed, and the task of the group understood. Table 5.2 outlines these phases.

Table 5.2 Tuckman's (1965) phases of group development

Phase	Characteristic	Effect on members	Outcome
Forming	Orientation, uncertainty, debate	Observing and testing out each other, looking for potential leaders and roles, become members or leaving group	Identification of common goals, early roles identified
Storming	Conflict, disputed control, anxiety, shifting identity	Disputes, challenges of roles, role change	Improved cohesion, trust, role definition and acceptance
Norming	Development of group identity and cohesion, practising and testing out group identity	Sense of belonging	Group rules established, focus on task of group
Performing	Goal-oriented activity, good morale	Individuals work for the group – committed to group rather than self	Able to work together to achieve goals
Adjourning	Closing down and reviewing of group identity and achievement	Reluctant to 'let go' of group identity, grieving processes	Group dispersed – individuals come to terms with loss of group role

These dynamics in group formation and working are often utilised by group facilitators when groups are important to achieving tasks. There is a **socialisation** process (Levine and Moreland, 1994) that translates the individual's identity to a social identity shared with the members of the group. Nurse education and training often follows these principles whereby a student gradually identifies with being a member of the nursing profession. A student nurse cohort will be encouraged to work in small groups on tasks to develop teamwork skills and develop this 'nurse' identity.

When groups go wrong

Table 5.1 outlines a good working group, but groups and teams can also be destructive and malfunctioning. What happens when individuals do not find a role or become the focus of blame for things going wrong, or when role conflict and disputes remain unresolved? The storming phase can continue or be re-visited in a group that does not gel well or is challenged by external forces. For example, when two people compete to be leader this can cause a split in the group and may result in a sub-group being formed.

When a group is challenged, stronger group members may find a weaker group member to blame and this individual becomes the **scapegoat** – the group adopts a belief that 'We'd be fine if it wasn't for John'.

For student groups to work well, Price (2003) suggests that members recognise that everyone will have a different contribution to make as inevitably some will be more knowledgeable and skilled than others. Roles will develop rather than be allocated, in recognition of members' diverse skills, but everyone has a role in collecting and disseminating learning. He suggests that a certain etiquette is helpful to the group process (Box 5.4).

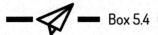 Box 5.4

Study group etiquette (after Price, 2003)

1   Roles of leader (chair) and group secretary should be rotated and shared.
2   Meetings should be arranged in advance.
3   Investigative roles should be shared.
4   Members should listen to each other without interruption.
5   Discussion needs to be constructive.
6   The group facilitator will control and re-direct the discussion.

Working groups can be disrupted when another member joins the group later, after the forming phase has occurred. This means the group must re-visit the forming stage to accommodate the new member. A well-formed and functioning group may have difficulty finding a role for the new member. Does this sound familiar? It is a typical experience in nursing training in practice areas. Let's see Box 5.5.

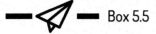 Box 5.5

Student experience of a group role

On an extended community placement, a third year student felt they had become a member of the team, with their own caseload and apparent acceptance as a valued contributor. The team decided to put staff photos on the wall to help patients feel welcomed. The team eagerly arranged a photo shoot and included everyone in the team including the cleaner and the community bus driver, but the student was not even considered for inclusion.

(Continued)

This student's role in the group as an equal member could not be accommodated in the minds of the group as it would otherwise threaten the existing group roles of the team, even though the student felt they was doing virtually the same job. The other team members saw the student role as temporary and not necessary for inclusion in the photo board of staff members who represented the stable and existing team.

Students often struggle to feel accepted and recognised for their contributions in the clinical area because the existing group has to maintain its own identity when the student is not there. Also, the group has to accommodate the student in a role that necessitates protection, tolerance and mentoring, something that doesn't apply to the rest of the team. The existing nursing team may have a 'reserved place' for someone in the role of pupil that is filled whenever a student arrives, but cannot afford to constantly re-visit the forming phase every time a new student arrives on the ward. After all, the existing nursing team is at the performing stage and the student has to fit in with an existing dynamic.

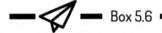 **Box 5.6**

Survival tip: the student in a nursing team

It is useful to remember group dynamics when joining a new nursing team in order to reduce the defensive reaction of the group. Remember, everyone already has a role in the team and you will provoke hostility if you encroach on those roles. The team will accommodate you but they will have preconceived expectations about what role you will take. You will do well to have good self-awareness, understand how you come across to others and be aware that this team will only allow a temporary role for you, because they have to function effectively when you are not there.

Group structures

Another way to look at groups is to consider the structures they form: the leadership hierarchy and communication channels between members. Families provide good examples of group structures because they tend not to change quickly over time. Let's look at some family structures.

Families tend to have clear hierarchies because usually the parents are in charge and the children only have power according to their ages and level of responsibility. Family therapist

Harry Wright suggests three types of structure which affect the flow of communication between members of a family (Wright, 1990).

The healthy hierarchy of a group (Figure 5.1) resembles a healthy family in which there is a clear delineation of responsibility but good communication channels.

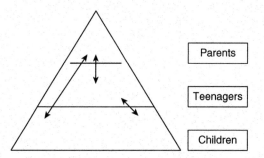

Figure 5.1 A healthy, democratic family structure

This type of structure is often called a **democratic leadership** style in which roles are well defined but all members have a say in the group's functions.

A rigid hierarchy has overbearing authoritarian leadership and poor or top-down communication channels. What the leadership say is what goes, with no argument!

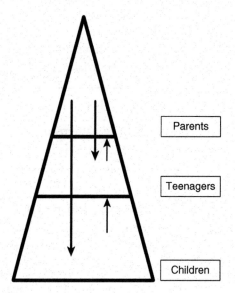

Figure 5.2 An authoritarian family structure

This is also known as an **authoritarian leadership** style in which the decision-makers are remote from the rest of the group and can cause frustration, disinterest and lack of motivation among group members.

The third type of hierarchy is a chaotic one: no one seems to be in charge and group members argue and do not work together; everyone has a say but no one is listening!

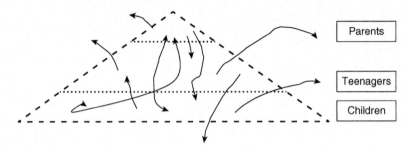

| Parents |
| Teenagers |
| Children |

Figure 5.3 A chaotic, laissez-faire family structure

This is referred to as a **laissez-faire leadership** (anything goes) style and tends to be characterised by lots of arguing but nothing getting done.

Lewin et al. (1939) famously studied these leadership styles and found that the most effective group structure and leadership style was the democratic one, with a leader who listens and discusses ideas with the group, but who also keeps control.

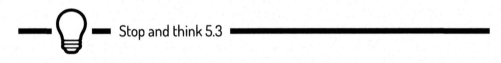

Stop and think 5.3

Have you ever experienced groups with these structures? How did you feel as a group member? Which one did you find most effective and enjoyable to be in and which one was most frustrating?

Families and work groups both show these patterns of group structure. Children in rigid families often have little sense of having someone to talk to about their problems – often an older sibling or a grandparent acts as the parental guide instead. Families with chaotic structures have chaotic dynamics; the parents lack authority, the children exhibit poor conduct and poor impulse control and even the family dog misbehaves! Groups and families with problematic leadership often exhibit disruptive communication channels. Let's look at some common patterns found in both families and work groups.

Scapegoating

As mentioned earlier, a group member can carry the problems of the group by being blamed for all its ills. An example could be when two people of equal status in a group can't agree but also can't blame each other for the stalemate. So, someone of a lesser status is blamed; two parents in marital difficulty may attribute their problems to a child's difficult behaviour or illness. The stress presented by the child acts as an excuse for the rift between the parents. Very often, however, it is the rift that has caused the child's misbehaviour or illness, which maintains the situation while the two parents ignore their own problems.

Triangulation

Triangulation can occur when two group members need a third member to intervene and sort out their conflict – a common dynamic involving someone who becomes 'the peace-maker'. In families a parent intervenes between two children, or a child may be compelled to intervene between two arguing parents.

Over-involvement

Over-involvement is over-protectiveness or interference of one member by another; often with a leader or peace-maker protecting someone put into the role of being 'vulnerable'. In families this is commonly a mother 'smothering' a child. In nurse training, this is seen commonly when a mentor is uncomfortable with allowing a student to take responsibility and is over-controlling of what the student does.

Dyads

A **dyad** is the communication pattern formed by two (or more) people who have made a small sub-group within a group, causing a bisection of the group. This is common in groups with a more rigid hierarchy, in which communication is not encouraged. It will happen in teaching groups when two students explain to each other what the teacher has just said, instead of asking for clarifiication from the teacher. We have all done this! In a family of authoritarian parents, children will form a dyad; a sub-group apart from the parents, creating an 'us and them' dynamic. In a work group, subordinate members (who may include students) will ally themselves with each other when communication with the authority figures is difficult, perhaps because of lack of time, or remoteness of the leaders.

Triads

A **triad** is a communication link that brings more than one opposing perspective to the group, causing a three-way split. This could be perhaps a parent and an older child both opposed to the other parent, or two or more siblings of different ages individually opposing a parent. Team members in divided work groups with remote and authoritarian leaders may create a triad where people are divided about how to deal with the leader; they argue between themselves and cut out the leader from the group dynamics. The leader then becomes more remote and distanced from the group.

Look at the vignette in Practice example box 5.1.

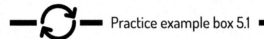 Practice example box 5.1

Example from practice

A mature second year student joined a medical ward's nursing team that was more accustomed to inexperienced, young, first year students. The mature student had worked as a healthcare assistant for many years, much longer than some of the younger qualified nurses had been in healthcare, and was highly competent with delivering hands-on care. The student started showing the ward healthcare assistants some of the 'tricks of the trade' and frequently talked about her experiences as a care assistant. The young mentor for this student found it difficult to teach the student anything because the student frequently said 'I know that'. The mentor started to get frustrated, the healthcare assistants withdrew and only talked among themselves and the other qualified nurses often gave the mentor knowing looks and sniggered when the mentor and student attempted any teaching interactions.

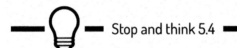 Stop and think 5.4

What group dynamics can you see occurring in Practice example box 5.1? Can you identify the possible patterns and roles in Table 5.3? Possible answers are given in Table 5.4.

Table 5.3 Group and communication dynamics

Question	Who?	Why?
Who forms dyads in this example?		
Who creates a triad?		
What is the result of this triad?		
Who is the leader?		
Who is likely to become isolated from the group?		

Table 5.4 Possible answers to Stop and think 5.4

Question	Who?	Why?
Who forms dyads in this example?	The healthcare assistants and the other qualified nurses.	To separate themselves from the conflict between the mentor and the student.
Who creates a triad?	The student, the mentor, the care assistants and the other nurses are all divided into sub-groups.	The care assistants feel threatened by the student, the other nurses distance themselves from the mentor and the student is shut out of both groups.
What is the result of this triad?	–	The working group is split into three sub-groups and one individual.
Who is the leader?	The mentor	The mentor is the one with the responsibility and power to change the situation.
Who is likely to become isolated from the group?	The student	The established group will normalise and the student will be scapegoated unless the mentor resolves the problem.

Groups and teams in practice

Professional groups

In the practice setting a student will join several different social groups and work teams. Socially, the student brings some group relationship factors to the practice area such as gender, age, ethnicity and cultural group identity. Also, the student will be placed in a pre-ordained group role such as 'student nurse'. The student will also categorise colleagues into groups such as 'doctor', 'nurse' and 'patient' as well as the social groups delineated by cultural perceptions of factors such as age, gender, ethnicity and level of authority. The student nurse, in joining professional groups, has to go through the process of forming, storming and norming in order to find a comfortable match between what they bring and what they are allowed to offer to the group.

Channels of communication will be more democratic in nursing teams generally, except those that have authoritarian leadership and fixed hierarchical structures. In these, unfortunately, the student may be quite low in the pecking order!

The multi-disciplinary team, however, presents a more rigid group overall. There is less opportunity for the student to assert their own character and assets to this team, and there will be a more powerful set of dynamics and identity already existing in this type of team to keep the status quo. Communication channels in multi-disciplinary teams are likely to vary depending on the structure of the group and leadership style. A strong and authoritarian medical consultant, for instance, will probably generate a top-down communication channel and only those close to the consultant in the hierarchy will have influence over group decisions. The student in these groups will need to communicate through the chain of command – through the mentor or ward manager – to get information across effectively. Multi-disciplinary teams with democratic structures will afford much more opportunity for the student to exercise assertiveness and contribute meaningfully to the group. The leader is likely to facilitate good communication channels while ensuring members of the group have equal say and do not engage in destructive dynamics such as forming sub-groups. See the practice example in Box 5.7.

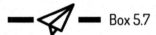 Box 5.7

An example of democratic leadership in CAMHS

A multi-disciplinary team meeting of a child and adolescent mental health service (CAMHS) team was led by a strong consultant psychiatrist and consisted of nurses, social workers, psychologists and occupational therapists. A newly qualified psychologist had recently joined the team and was rather over-enthusiastic about their own abilities. During a clinical meeting, they frequently interrupted the nurses who were giving their assessment and recommendations for a young patient. The consultant allowed some of these interruptions but eventually reminded the psychologist that all professional assessments would be heard, including theirs, and that the nurses' assessment was particularly important as they had spent a whole week with this patient, whereas others had only had an hour at a time to assess the different aspects of his needs.

The psychologist kept quiet and others in the team looked at each other in relief that the psychologist had finally been put in their place!

Patient groups: families

Patients bring their group identities and roles with them into healthcare settings. They too are socioculturally linked to gender, age, class and ethnicity groups and they also have occupational, social and family group identities. Patients' families often demonstrate powerful group dynamics when the patient is ill; the health problem is often a challenge to the equilibrium of their family. The patient's role in the family is likely to change due to their illness and vulnerability. Other family members will take on roles of protectors, leaders or decision-makers. Thus, the patient's family as a group re-visits the storming and norming phases of the group process. Television programmes set in hospitals often relish portraying the storming aspects of families suddenly in dispute because of an accident or illness of one of its members. There are usually dramatic bedside scenes involving family members arguing and then resolving their problems. Although fictional, it reflects in dramatic style the turbulence that families experience when the group is threatened by illness. As nurses, our role is likely to be protection and care for the patient but, in recognising the holistic needs of the patient, our attention should also be on the family. We should consider how they are coping with the challenges presented by both the illness and the possibility of family members having to take on a caring role in the longer-term. See case study in Box 5.8.

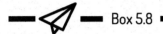 Box 5.8

Case study of family dynamics and communication

An older man with Alzheimer's disease was admitted to hospital for assessment following concerns over his physical wellbeing. He lived alone with a daughter nearby and a son some distance away. It was found that this man would need 24-hour care to maintain his safety. His daughter did not want to disrupt family life for her children by having her father living with her, but felt guilty about refusing to offer to be his carer. Her brother did not want to get involved as he lived on his own and had a career, but he too felt guilty about being unsupportive and insensitive. The nurse heard from both relatives independently about how they were feeling. They did not want to share their anxieties with the other and thus be more of a burden to each other. The nurse facilitated a meeting between the brother and sister to talk about their feelings together and they resolved to share the care. The brother had the financial means to fund a care home place near his sister and she could visit regularly and ensure their father was well cared for.

The case study outlines a very typical scenario involving a family adjusting to a relative in need. Dementia often challenges families to engage in role reversal, as the traditional head of the family becomes dependent and the children become the decision-makers. Where several adult children are concerned there is often a degree of storming as they adjust to new roles between themselves.

Patient groups: clinical applications

Groups can be powerful tools for changing how people see themselves and for gaining a social identity. You may have already found that your personal self-confidence has changed if you have developed a social identity as a nurse. The power of groups is also effective in changing how patients see themselves, improving self-esteem and empowering patients to be more assertive. For instance, people recovering from substance-use problems gain a social identity of being 'in recovery' when identifying with mutual aid groups such as Alcoholics Anonymous, and this enables them to remain abstinent and protects against relapse (Best et al., 2016; Mawson et al., 2015).

Groups are used extensively in mental health practice to support patients' self-esteem, behaviour change and social skills (for example, Pollard and Cook, 2012; Sturgeon et al., 2018). Also, groupwork has effective application for health promotion and psychosocial wellbeing for a range of patient groups including older people (Haslam et al., 2010), adults with learning difficulties (Marwood and Hewitt, 2016) and parents of young patients (Popplestone-Helm and Helm, 2009).

Other patient groups include educative and health promotion groups, perhaps run by community and outpatient nurses as a group clinic. Such groups may be convened to help patients with similar health problems to come to terms with managing their condition and learning from the facilitator and each other to cope with their health status and its implications. These groups might include a group for newly diagnosed patients with type 2 diabetes, where the group's aims will be healthier eating, monitoring and compliance with health regimes. Another common educative patient group may be an obesity clinic, for adults or children, a smoking-cessation group in a GP surgery or a supportive group for informal carers of patients with dementia or learning difficulties. Each group will have its own aims but these often include meeting motivational, educational and self-esteem needs among members.

Conclusion

This chapter has provided a brief overview of a large body of evidence around group dynamics, group communication and the effect and application of group dynamics among professional and patient groups. For the student nurse, a major task is simply coping with the frequent changes in group membership that goes with changing clinical practice placements and coping with being a temporary member of existing teams. This task is difficult and should not be underestimated by students, mentors or tutors. However, as training progresses and confidence, self-awareness and assertiveness skills develop, the student nurse will soon be able to take these challenges in their stride and use the opportunities to develop teamwork skills that will be necessary in their future nursing practice.

FURTHER READING

Bach, S. and Ellis, P. (2018) *Leadership, Management and Team Working in Nursing (Transforming Nursing Practice Series)*. London, Learning Matters (SAGE).

REFERENCES

Asch, S. (1955) Opinions and social pressures. *Scientific American*, 193, 31–55.
Belbin, R. (1981) *Management Teams: Why They Succeed or Fail*. Oxford, Butterworth-Heinemann.

Benne, K. and Sheats, P. (1948) Functional roles of group members. *Journal of Social Issues*, 4, 41–49.

Best, D., Beckwith, M., Haslam, C., Haslam, S.A., Jetten, J., Mawson, E. and Lubman, D.I. (2016) Overcoming alcohol and other drug addiction as a process of social identity transition: the social identity model of recovery (SIMOR). *Addiction Research & Theory*, 24(2), 111–123.

Haslam, C., Haslam, S.A., Jetten, J., Bevins, A., Ravenscroft, S. and Tonks, J. (2010) The social treatment: the benefits of group interventions in residential care settings. *Psychology and Aging*, 25(1), 157–167.

Jackson, D., Hickman, L., Power, T., Disler, R., Potgieter, I., Deek, H. and Davidson, P. (2014) Small group learning: graduate health students' views of challenges and benefits. *Contemporary Nurse*, 48(1), 117–128.

Levine, J. and Moreland, R. (1994) Group socialization: theory and research. *European Review of Social Psychology*, 5(1), 305–336.

Lewin, K., Lippitt, R. and White, R. (1939) Patterns of aggressive behaviour in experimentally created 'social climates'. *Journal of Experimental Psychology*, 4(1), 19–31.

Marwood, H. and Hewitt, O. (2016) Evaluating an anxiety group for people with learning disabilities using a mixed methodology. *British Journal of Learning Disabilities*, 41, 150–158.

Mawson, E., Best, D., Beckwith, M., Dingle, G.A. and Lubman, D.I. (2015) Social identity, social networks and recovery capital in emerging adulthood: a pilot study. *Substance Abuse Treatment, Prevention, and Policy*, 10, 45.

NMC (2018) *The Code: Professional Standards of Practice and Behaviour for Nurses, Midwives and Nursing Associates*. www.nmc.org.uk/standards/code/.

Pollard, N. and Cook, S. (2012) The power of low-key groupwork activities in mental health support work. *Groupwork*, 22(3), 7–32.

Popplestone-Helm, S.V. and Helm, D.P. (2009) Setting up a support group for children and their well carers who have a significant adult with a life-threatening illness. *International Journal of Palliative Nursing*, 5(5), 214–221.

Price, B. (2003) *Studying Nursing Using Problem-Based & Enquiry-Based Learning*. Basingstoke, Palgrave Macmillan.

Punshon, G., Endacott, R., Aslett, P., Brocksom, J., Fleure, L., Howdle, F., O'Connor, A., Swift, A., Trevatt, P. and Leary, A. (2017) The experiences of specialist nurses working within the uro-oncology multidisciplinary team in the United Kingdom. *Clinical Nurse Specialist*, 31(4), 210–218.

Sherif, M., Harvey, O., White, B., Hood, W. and Sherif, C. (1961) *Intergroup Conflict and Cooperation; The Robber's Cave Experiment*. Norman, OK, University of Oklahoma.

Sturgeon, M., Tylera, N. and Gannon, T. (2018) A systematic review of group work interventions in UK high secure hospitals. *Aggression and Violent Behavior*, 38, 53–75.

Tajfel, H. and Turner, J. (1979) An integrative theory of intergroup conflict. In G. Austin and S. Worchel (eds), *The Social Psychology of Intergroup Relations* (pp. 33–47). Monterey, CA, Brooks/Cole.

Tuckman, B. (1965) Development sequence in small groups. *Psychological Bulletin*, 63, 384–399.

Wright, H. (1990) *Groupwork*. London, Scutari Press.

SIX
EFFECTIVE PERSON-CENTRED AND INTERCULTURAL COMMUNICATION

GAYATRI NAMBIAR-GREENWOOD AND SARAH RUTHERFORD

....THIS CHAPTER WILL HELP YOU TO:

- Engage with people from diverse communities and backgrounds
- Recognise factors that lead to unconscious bias
- Challenge preconceptions that interfere with effective communication
- Develop cultural self-awareness

Introduction

This chapter sees all communication, even between people who may appear to share obvious characteristics such as the same ethnicity or nationality, as intercultural communication. The aim of this chapter is to raise awareness about how unintended, unconscious bias can influence two-way communication between health professionals and their patients.

Discussions around intercultural communication tend to focus on conversations or difficulties of communicating with people whose culture differs from the Western ideas of cultural norms. However, culture is not limited to ethnicity or race but consists of a wide variety of factors that influence our thinking, ideas, prejudices and level of comfort when conversing with those outside our known communities. In a healthcare setting, this can affect an individual's access to an equal share of services.

It is important to note that culture is not solely the experience of patients but that the intercultural experiences of healthcare professionals equally impact on the effectiveness of communication.

Therefore, this chapter discusses culture and intercultural communication based on the premise that all people are cultural beings, whatever their ethnicity, illness, ability, disability, gender, sexuality or profession.

The context of intercultural communication

In order to broaden the discussion and encourage intercultural communication as a way of promoting equality, the chapter adopts the definition of culture by the medical anthropologist, Cecil Helman (2007:4):

> a set of inherited guidelines (explicit and implicit) which as members of a certain society inform us how to view our world and how to experience it emotionally ... [that determines] ... how we behave in it, in relation to others, to our understanding of supernatural forces or gods and to our natural environment ... [and that it provides us with the] ... symbols, language, art and literature that we transmit to the next generation ... as a form of preservation of that cultural identity.

This chapter adopts this broad definition because it argues culture is not limited to individuals or groups of a certain ethnicity. It transcends ethnicity and includes sexuality, gender and disability, among others. An individual's life is made up of a number of factors that intersect and affect their perspective (see Figure 6.1). As health professionals we must pay attention to the diverse needs of the patient and treat them in a way that works towards equitable delivery of healthcare.

Additionally, the NMC *Code* (NMC, 2018) states that nurses should ensure that those receiving care are 'treated with respect, that their rights are upheld and that any discriminatory attitudes and behaviours towards those receiving care are challenged'.

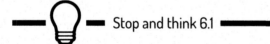 Stop and think 6.1

If you met a group of young unemployed men, from diverse ethnic backgrounds, but from the same low-income area, they may share an accent and have had the same educational journey. However, they may have different reasons and personal experiences as to why they left school early, did not go to college, do not have a job or are not employable. Change their gender and again the reasons will be different.

Their personal experiences create varying aspects of their culture: perhaps how their parents socialised them, where they live, who are their friends, the sports and teams they support or whom they may see as responsible for their present status (positively or negatively) could be among many more reasons. These various factors, resulting in very individual cultural stories, are referred to as **intersectionality** (see Figure 6.1). So, if they become ill and hospitalised, their main concern might not be their culture or religious practice but other factors that may appear more pressing at that point.

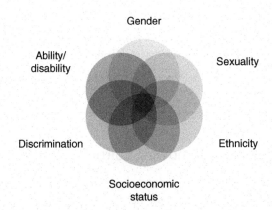

Figure 6.1   Intersections of factors that determine an individual's culture

Books on communication often provide health and social care staff with tips and ways to improve interactions with patient or clients. While this guidance is useful and effective at a general level, intercultural communication aims to enhance communication so that we meet the individual needs of clients and patients and provide person-centred care. It requires that the health and social care professional appreciates that all individuals have cultural needs, even if they are not immediately obvious, and especially when they may look, speak or express themselves exactly like the nurse.

The NMC (2018) states that we are required to treat people as individuals and uphold their dignity, among others, by treating people with kindness, respect and compassion, avoiding assumptions and recognising diversity and individual choice in our patients.

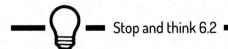 Stop and think 6.2

While in practice, you see a white British woman, who has come in for a laparoscopy, approach a healthcare assistant (HCA). She says she does not like sharing the bay with men she does not know and asks to be moved. She has just seen the HCA move an Asian woman to another bay, with just women patients. The HCA sighs and walks away, saying that she needs to speak

(Continued)

to the nurse-in-charge about this. The HCA tells you later that she feels annoyed because the patient does not have any obvious religious reasons to be moved. Consider these questions:

1   Why do you think the HCA did not consider the patient's personal needs to be as pressing as those of the Asian woman?
2   What do you think the patient may have perceived when the HCA sighed and needed to speak to someone in greater authority at the request to be moved?

Possible answer: clearly the judgement about cultural need is based on visual cues and assumptions about ethnicity, but without taking into account any cultural differences between the women. The patient may well have interpreted the reaction by the HCA as discrimination based on an assumption that she does not have any claim to religious or cultural grounds for preference.

Influences on our ways of knowing culture

Culture is affected by external factors such as history, politics and media. They are considered the dominant influencers of the culture we choose to associate with (Papastergiadis, 2013). These dominant influencers affect our understanding of who we are, which groups we identify with in society and the values we see as significant. The culture of an individual or group is never a static experience. It is sometimes overtly obvious, but mainly subtle. It changes, modifies and adapts over time by being influenced at a personal level, genetically and socially.

The aspect of cultural self-identity that an individual chooses to identify with is selected interchangeably. For example, your identity may be as a health professional at work but with your friends you may adopt an alternative persona and even an altered style of language. At different points, you reflect a variety of values to adapt to the situation. Among others' identities, we modify our labels from a social, psychological and ethnic perspective, portraying a persona as a confident or shy person, and with gender or class labels at the same time. Therefore, you could refer to yourself as a male nurse in one situation and as a middle-class man in another.

Everyday political, mass media and historical conversations regarding culture tend to focus on black and ethnic minority (BAME) populations and their differences from a collective, or 'us', mainly comparing BAME populations to the majority population. These types of portrayal also tend to limit the diverse cultures of many large populations to a single stereotyped group, claiming they all share one culture. This overlooks the diverse needs of all populations and makes assumptions about the cultural differences between BAME individuals.

The multi-layering of politics, mass media and social media has an echo-chamber effect where we tend to listen, read and engage with people, newspapers and social media that support our view, separating us from trying to listen, consider or empathise with another's perspective. This can contribute to either over-identifying with a culture or alienation from those we see as a cultural other. In addition, due to the persistence of stigma and derogatory labels from external sources, individuals and communities can, over time, internalise and adopt the negative self-identities assigned to them.

Figure 6.2 provides one interconnected example of how perspectives of history, politics and media, which may not be factually correct, can influence how we see others at a personal and societal level.

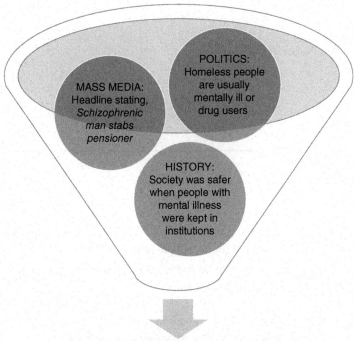

PERSONAL: You harbour fears of being assaulted by someone who is homeless. You start questioning whether homeless people should be in institutions.

Figure 6.2 Interconnected influencers

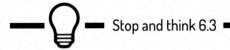 Stop and think 6.3

See Table 6.1 and think about your own diversity characteristics (age, gender, social class, social circumstances, economic status, regional background, accent and so on). Consider the stereotypes applied to your characteristics and decide the degree, on a scale of 1–10, to which they represent you. The first row is completed as an example.

(Continued)

Use the last box to reflect on how this stereotype makes you feel.

Table 6.1 Personal characteristics

Characteristic	Stereotype	How like me is this?
Example: Quiet young Muslim woman who wears a hijab, attends clinic with husband	She is probably oppressed	3
Reflect on how the stereotype(s) may make you feel		

Authority

At times, a patient or client may hesitate, be scared or limit their conversation with us due to previous experiences of talking to people who they perceive to be in authority. A few examples of how unconscious (or, at times, conscious) authority can affect the communication between nurses and patients are:

- the status and role of the patient, in comparison to the professional
- the perceived attitude of the healthcare team with regard to the group of which the patient is thought to be part (gender, age, tribe, class, sexual orientation, cause of admission)
- the ability to speak a certain language or the ability to formulate and express oneself easily, logically and emotionally.

Some examples of how assumptions about authority can affect healthcare are given in Table 6.2.

Table 6.2 Examples of how authority can influence care provision

Patient or professional status/ authority	Cultural and authority assumptions	Impact on care delivered
A senior health professional admitted as a patient	They're cleverer than me and already know what to do about their condition Worry about giving the wrong information	May be avoided by health or social care staff Minimal care delivered Inadequate information being shared

Patient with limited English	They are not able to understand anything The information needs to be given to family members who understand the language better	Health and social care staff provide minimal information Issues of confidentiality may be breached Impatience at times Patient will not feel able to question care or ask for specific treatment
Asylum seeker	They may be worried that their application will be affected if they do not comply with care Seen as socially and possibly educationally inferior Should be grateful for the support provided	The patient/service user will not ask for services they need or seek clarifications about service provision Reluctance to draw attention to service failings Care not explained or choices offered Impatient or irritated when they are not grateful for the care received
Person with Down's syndrome	Has a learning disability Unable to understand information Is 'sweet'	Inadequate information is provided. Family and carers given information first or instead of the service user Choices not offered

Limitations or barriers to effective intercultural communication

We have implied that communication focuses on the ways in which nurses should talk to patients of different cultures, but it is also important to note that effective communication is a reciprocal, two-way experience. The nurse needs to be aware (and self-aware) that there may be unconscious elements of themselves that inhibit and limit the extent to which the patient chooses to disclose or share.

Table 6.3 refers to the more common areas and concepts that occur unintentionally within us that can inhibit intercultural communication. Consider your thoughts and what actions you could take if you encounter these scenarios during your practice.

Table 6.3 Common areas and concepts of unconscious bias

Common areas and concepts of unconscious bias	Examples
The cultural 'other': this notion comes from an imagined idea of difference, either superior or inferior, to the cultural self-identity or social identities that may represent the norm. In childhood, identifying with the cultural 'other' is a natural process of choice but as an adult the process of constructing or perpetuating a cultural 'other' can be intensified by unfounded subjective feelings of insecurity and helplessness.	A woman from a traveller family has been admitted and she has a large family who, despite being advised, visit her in large numbers at all times of the day. They do not seem to understand when you tell them she is very ill and needs rest. There is a woman who has been admitted from a detention centre for illegal migrants. She is waiting to be returned to her country of origin. She eats a specific diet as a religious observance. Some of your team make no effort and provide her with a very basic, monotonous diet as they feel she should not have been in the country anyway.

(Continued)

Table 6.3 (Continued)

Common areas and concepts of unconscious bias	Examples
Unconscious bias: sometimes referred to as a 'blink of the eye', or aversive or unintentional discrimination. Such unconscious biases lead to unthinking ways of discriminating against others and can even be invisible to those who perpetrate it.	White male physicians who are less likely to prescribe pain medication to black men than to white men, due to the assumption of drug abuse among black men.
	Doctors and nurse assume their low-income patients are less intelligent, more likely to engage in risky behaviours and less likely to adhere to health advice.
	Pregnant women face discrimination from healthcare providers on the basis of their ethnicity and socioeconomic background.
	Women presenting with cardiac heart disease symptoms are significantly less likely than men to receive diagnosis, referral and treatment, due to misdiagnosis of stress/anxiety.
Ethnocentrism: a state comparable to racism or the foundation of racism, where one believes that one's culture or cultural facet is the superior or the best culture. Ethnocentrism is judging another culture, negatively and solely by the values and standards of one's own culture. It is one of the foundations for racism.	A child is born to a South Asian family with severe disabilities. An assumption is made that the parents are closely related.
	The priority of those from the deaf community is integration into the majority or hearing community.
	A nurse specialist does not put forward the names of patients from a certain low-income area for a drug trial as she feels that they are not interested in participating in the study.
Intercultural communication apprehension: the fear or anxiety, real or imaginary, associated with anticipated communication with people from different groups, especially different cultural and/or ethnic groups. Politics, media and history often perpetuate this. Political correctness is often blamed for this.	Nursing staff avoid interacting with a transgender man and put him in side room.
	Midwives avoid asking African immigrants about female genital mutilation experiences and expectations because of uncertainty about how to address such cultural practices.
	Nurses provide all patients from South Asian backgrounds a halal diet without question, so that they do not offend them.

Challenges of cultural self-awareness

The starting point of becoming self-aware about unconscious bias is admitting we all experience it. Papadopoulos (2011) feels that this self-awareness can crucially contribute towards our understanding of how we construct and see ourselves and others who are different from us.

Neuliep (2015) states that this examination of self-identity can positively influence issues around intercultural communication apprehension and reduce ethnocentricity. However, dealing with our own unconscious bias is more than just engaging in compulsory online courses on equality and diversity. These online exercises do not take into account that completing a tool about being fair to those labelled differently can simply add to intercultural communication apprehension. There is also the possibility that such exercises, without space for discussion, is continuing to frame intercultural communication as not normal.

Engaging in self-awareness, however, can be an uncomfortable exercise for anyone, as it requires us to be honest about our previous errors, ethnocentricities and personally held prejudices. Health and social care professionals with a lack of self-awareness about their own ethnocentric views or paternalistic attitudes can immediately stifle the communication process and stop it from being a mutually beneficial experience. Knowing our own strengths and limitations, understanding our own emotions and the impact of our behaviour in diverse situations serves to enhance therapeutic relationships with others in any healthcare setting.

Language

How we use language verbally and non-verbally can demonstrate cultural inclusivity or division. This can include the terminology used to describe different groups and communities. Words and terms that a cultural group regard as derogatory or demeaning can be alienating, with resulting adverse outcomes for care delivery. Examples of this might be terms used to describe the BAME population, the pronouns used for transgender and non-binary individuals and how we describe disability.

For example, describing someone as being 'a schizophrenic' implies that this is a personal characteristic. Describing them as 'an individual with schizophrenia' recognises that their condition is an external condition but is not intrinsic to who they are. This labelling can apply to all diseases or conditions (e.g. 'diabetic', 'autistic', 'depressive', 'dementia patient') and reduces the person to being labelled by their condition or disability.

Evidence of healthcare professionals understanding cultural language preferences indicates a respect for that group or individual.

Non-native speakers of English and non-verbal patients

Patients for whom English is not their first language, and those who are unable to verbalise any language, can experience significant social isolation and disempowerment in an environment where they are unable to express themselves effectively.

In this instance, it is imperative that nurses and all health and social care professionals empathise and make efforts to ensure that people are not ignored and overlooked. In these instances, the verbal communication takes second place to the non-verbal communication and sensitive interpersonal skills. Here, the recipient of care will be paying greater attention to these factors, to elicit whether or not the nurse will invest time and effort in their care for them.

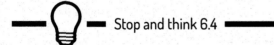 Stop and think 6.4

Below are inter-related functions of non-verbal communication. Think of the times you may have used this in communicating with patients or clients.

(Continued)

1 Non-verbal communication can simply be to reinforce a verbal message, for example pointing to a medication, and the action of lifting a cup to your mouth, as a way of taking their medication with a drink. The purpose in this context is to increase the likelihood of the accurate reception of the verbal message.

2 Non-verbal communication can be a substitute for a verbal message. For instance, waving or beckoning can be used where verbal communication is sub-optimal due to distance or other situational factors.

3 The third function is to emphasise a verbal message, for instance pausing before speaking, touching or leaning forward, sighing or rolling your eyes while talking or simply saying something louder.

4 Non-verbal signals can also contradict the verbal message. For example, a flat tone of voice, fixed facial expression or lack of eye contact can undermine any positive verbal expression or apology.

5 Generally, non-verbal messages can adjust the process of social intercourse by indicating that it is someone else's turn to speak or that a conversation is ending or entering a new phase. For some communities or individuals with forms of altered cognition (forms of learning disability, dementia or cognitive deficits) non-verbal messages may be misinterpreted.

Developing cultural self-awareness to improve intercultural communication

As mentioned in Chapter 2, the use of self-awareness tools such as the Johari window can be a starting place to work through and challenge the assumptions we all hold. Table 6.4 is a reminder of the areas of your own self-awareness; this time, focus on how you see yourself, your culture and those who are different from you.

Table 6.4 The Johari window

	Known to self	Not known to self
Known to others	Open area	Blind area
Not known to others	Hidden area	Unknown area

Source: Luft, 1969

Another exercise that can be utilised to consider self-awareness, either individually or in groups, is Cultural Circles (adapted from Coombs and Sarason, 1998). Answer the questions below by yourself, or with a group of colleagues, taking turns to answer each one. The exercise will encourage you to recognise yourself as a cultural person.

1 Describe your cultural background. Other than your ethnicity, try to focus on what distinguishes you culturally from people you consider the same and different from you. You can define your culture in as narrow or as broad terms as you like.

2 Of what aspects of your cultural background are you most proud? (This can include personal, familial or national factors.)

Conclusion

All communication is intercultural communication. In an increasingly diverse and globalised world, healthcare professionals need to reconsider their definitions of culture and those factors that influence their perspectives and preconceptions. Without developing a self-awareness around the interactions with those whom we do not consider to be like ourselves, our inherent unconscious biases and apprehensions have the ability to limit, challenge and offend individuals in our professional care. Fostering cultural self-awareness is not without challenges but lays the foundation for person-centred, individualised care.

REFERENCES

Coombs, G. and Sarason, Y. (1998) Culture circles: a cultural self-awareness exercise. *Journal of Management Education*, 22(2), 218–226.

Helman, C.G. (2007) *Culture, Health and Illness* (5th edn). London, Hodder Arnold.

Luft, J. (1969) *Of Human Interaction*. Palo Alto, CA, National Press Books.

Neuliep, J.W. (2015) Uncertainty and anxiety in intercultural encounters. *The International Encyclopedia of Interpersonal Communication*, 1–9.

NMC (2018) *The Code: Professional Standards of Practice and Behaviour for Nurses, Midwives and Nursing Associates*. www.nmc.org.uk/standards/code/.

Papadopoulos, I. (2011) Courage, compassion and cultural competence. In *The 13th Anna Reynvaan Lecture*, 19 May 2011, Amsterdam, Netherlands.

Papastergiadis, N. (2013) *The Turbulence of Migration: Globalization, Deterritorialization and Hybridity* (2nd edn). Cambridge, Polity Press.

PART II
APPLYING COMMUNICATION SKILLS IN NURSING

Preface to Part 2

The first section of this book focused particularly on the basic theories of communication, giving you the underpinning concepts and philosophies that support communication skills and knowledge.

Part 2 now builds on that basis by examining how the theory is applied in the practice setting. It begins by examining the application of the basic skills, demonstrating the theory–practice bridge in different but common fields of nursing care (Chapter 7). In every field of nursing there are specific challenges in delivering care that reflect the wider socioeconomic and political contexts that structure care (Chapter 8).

Currently we are faced with an ageing global population and the challenge that living with chronic conditions can present. Healthcare policies globally are turning to health promotion and encouraging greater self-care to improve the health of populations and to encourage self-management of challenges such as diabetes or learning difficulty (Chapter 9). We are also facing unprecedented human mobility in the modern era that presents challenges of cultural differences in health beliefs, histories and expectations. The NMC charges nurses and midwives to meet these challenges by becoming more adept at communicating health promotion (Chapter 10), empowering people towards autonomous care and managing effectively the communication needs of diverse groups, communities and individuals.

Part 2 will explore these challenges and describe and explore how we can use communication skills to meet these needs.

SEVEN
THEORY TO PRACTICE: COMMUNICATING THERAPEUTICALLY

EULA MILLER AND LUCY WEBB

.... THIS CHAPTER WILL HELP YOU TO:

- Demonstrate empathy and develop trusting nurse–patient relationships
- Empower people to meet their own needs and make choices
- Act professionally to ensure that personal judgements, prejudices, values, attitudes and beliefs do not compromise care
- Use helpful and therapeutic strategies to enable people to understand treatments

Introduction

In this chapter the aim is to identify fundamental approaches in therapeutic communication in modern nursing practice and link them to practice-based care. This chapter will focus on two specific paradigms of interaction pertinent to nursing care communication. These are the humanistic, or person-centred, approach and the cognitive-behavioural, or behaviour-change-centred, approach. First, we will look at person-centred approaches.

Person-centred communication

Chapter 4 looked at the nurse–patient relationship and emphasised the importance of developing a caring partnership between the nurse and the patient. Theories of modern nursing care and the nurse–patient relationship indicate that the essential components of the relationship are humanistic caring (Adams, 2016). The NMC (2018) describes person-centred care as:

an approach where the person is at the centre of the decision-making processes and the design of their care needs, their nursing care and treatment plan.

(NMC, 2018:39)

This approach recognises that the person is uniquely placed to experience their world and their own needs, while the practitioner's role is to validate that experience and help the person interpret it more effectively. The humanistic approach is often termed person-centred for the very reason that the person is seen as the 'expert' and has a unique perspective of their care needs and illness management. Many counselling styles are structured around this approach and one of its key theorists and exponents was Carl Rogers.

Rogerian counselling: the three core conditions of non-directive therapy

Carl Rogers (1961) was a psychotherapist who devised what is probably the most commonly used method of counselling and active listening in the health, social care and education fields. It adopts the humanistic preconcepts of adaptive development as encapsulated in **Maslow's hierarchy of needs** (Maslow, 1970), which holds that human development always strives to allow a person to become all that one can be. Rogers' **client-centred therapy** is based on the principle that the therapy is **non-directive**. The relationship is one of equals: the client (not 'patient') is able to grow and develop given suitable conditions and the practitioner's role gives **empowerment** to the client so that they can reach their human potential.

The three conditions are:

1   **Warmth and genuineness** on the part of the practitioner, in that they are genuinely interested and personally engaged in the process. This means the practitioner cannot get away with a superficial pretence of caring. The practitioner needs to be genuinely concerned for the client.
2   **Empathy** from the practitioner, who is able to relate to the person's experience. This is empathy as opposed to sympathy. The practitioner needs to be able to understand the person's experience, but not necessarily agree with their interpretation of it.
3   **Unconditional positive regard** from the practitioner in accepting the validity and value of the person's experiences. This also demands a division between accepting the person's views without necessarily agreeing with them. In fact, it is the difference between the practitioner's view and the client's view that often demonstrates the difference between coping and not coping. Therefore, the practitioner needs to have a more adaptive approach to the problem than the client.

In a nursing context the humanistic approach compliments holistic care in that it recognises patient uniqueness and supports individualised care. It could be said that the nurse's role is to translate best practice evidence from what works for groups of patients to what will work for a particular person: Mrs Smith or Mr Jones. To do this, the nurse is helped by models that structure the nurse–patient interaction.

Structuring the nurse–patient encounter

Boundaries of time, depth and mutuality

A therapeutic process involving a practitioner and a patient is described by Murray Cox (1978) as being structured by time, depth and mutuality. By this, he means that the structure of the interaction can be controlled by these three boundaries. Time refers to the limit of the length of the encounter, depth refers to the degree of seriousness and involvement of the material being addressed and mutuality refers to the degree of shared personal psychological contact, or engagement, entered into by the practitioner and the patient. These boundaries define the nature and the quality of the relationship and indicate what is therapeutic and what is not. Let us deal with some key elements to these boundaries in a nursing context.

Time

When an interaction is short it is difficult to convey the seriousness of the attention we want to give our patients. With a seriously ill or upset person, we may feel the need to give them all the time they may want. This is not always practical, nor indeed necessary or therapeutic. It is therefore important to tell the person how much time we can give them so that they know how to 'use' us.

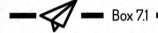 Box 7.1

The nervous patient

A man due to have open heart surgery is ready for his operation but has not yet had his sedating medication. He is experiencing anxiety about the operation. He asks the nurse to repeat the explanation of what will happen during the operation. She doesn't have much time but recognises that he is anxious. She gives him a sympathetic look and tells him she can spare 5 minutes. She asks what it is that is really bothering him. He gives it some thought, looks embarrassed, and says, 'I think it's the procedure itself – what would happen if I woke up with my chest opened up?' She smiles and gives him an explanation of what the anaesthetist does to monitor the patient. She says he won't be aware of anything until he wakes up in the post-operative recovery room where he will be monitored by a nurse. The man appears reassured.

In Box 7.1 the patient appears to be worried about the procedure. The nurse is busy but recognises that his need is important. The nurse structures this time for the patient by simply stating she has 5 minutes. This may sound a bit abrupt, but the patient then knows that he needs to focus on what his real worries are. Have you ever noticed that people often blurt out something important at the last minute, just before you have to leave? By stating the time limit, the nurse indicates to the patient that they need to address the 'burning issue', whatever it is.

When time is abundant or the patient very needy, time structuring is also important. A needy patient can demand attention and use time ineffectively. The nurse can use time structure to effect better communication, for instance by stating when and for how long the interaction will take place. The needy patient is then more likely to focus on the issues and use the time effectively.

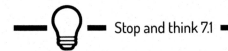 Stop and think 7.1

When you next go on placement (or when thinking about your last placement), consider how the healthcare staff around you use time with patients effectively but therapeutically. Do effective staff members use certain phrases? Make a note of them and discuss with your practice supervisor which ones would be appropriate, therapeutic and effective for you to use.

Depth

Depth is the degree of disclosure and the amount of investment the patient and the nurse are making. A therapeutic interaction, for Cox (1978), always moves towards disclosure of material. Cox divides disclosure of material in the therapeutic encounter into three stages, with one leading to the next:

Unconscious → conscious-withheld → conscious-disclosed

In Box 7.1, the nurse aids the patient in exploring what is troubling him (what is in his unconscious). By this he is led to his own realisation of what the problem is (conscious-withheld) and then reveals it to the nurse and so 'owns' it (conscious-disclosed). He perhaps didn't know at first what the problem was (unconscious), then he realised he was scared of waking up and felt ashamed of admitting it (conscious-withheld), but through the empathy of the nurse, 'owned up' to his fear and received reassurance.

Depth can also be divided into levels of disclosure. Cox (1978) calls these:

First level (trivial): 'I see it is raining again.'

Second level (neutral-personal): 'I don't like it raining all the time.'

Third level (emotional-personal): 'The rain reminds me of my father's funeral.'

The first level of disclosure is just interpersonal chat, but it does start a conversation and opens up opportunities for greater disclosure. The second is disclosure that is about the person, but has no emotional content. The person is disclosing a thought or opinion, but it is not personally important. The third, however, is both personal and emotional. There is emotional investment in the statement and often, for Cox, at a level that would not be revealed in a 'normal' conversation, and may be something revealed for the very first time. It could be regarded as a privilege to be given such trust by someone who makes a third-level disclosure to us.

Mutuality

The nurse–patient relationship is one made up of two people in alliance, with the aim of solving the patient's health-related problems. Cox (1978) describes mutuality as referring to:

how much the [practitioner] discloses about himself in order to share with the patient the experience he is disclosing.

(Cox, 1978:170)

In other words, the nurse cannot hide entirely behind a professional façade and not also be a 'person' to the patient. However, by 'disclosure' Cox is not referring to sharing stories of experiences. We cannot, as nurses, share our life experience directly with our patients. We might not know what it is like to be diagnosed with a serious illness. But we can put ourselves, personally, into the person's shoes and accept what they describe as their experience. Mutuality can look like an applied form of empathy in which it is not enough to simply empathise.

Mutuality is easier to apply to someone we like than when we cannot relate to the other person's experience or values. Cox gives an excellent example of this. In his work with psychopathic patients in Broadmoor Hospital in the UK he was often challenged by a lack of ability to relate to the patients' direct experiences. He describes maintaining the therapeutic space of mutuality with one patient by adopting a framework for the interaction as:

One of us is a rapist.

(Cox, 1978:169)

We could translate this therapeutic space of mutuality in the nurse–patient relationship as:

One of us has terminal cancer.

or

One of us is going home at the end of the shift.

This framework helps the nurse identify their 'position' with the patient which enables the two people to discuss the issues. The nurse does not have to be able to say 'I know how you feel'. However, the nurse can say, 'I hear your experience and accept it without interpretation or judgement'. Mutuality is the genuine collaboration of two people who, while very different, can work together as human beings to address the patient's problems.

Time, depth and mutuality work together to structure a therapeutic interaction or professional relationship. These three dimensions help us map a relationship and evaluate its effectiveness. However, it is important that the practitioner has good self-awareness. For nurses, this may be a challenge unless personal and professional development are valued in the clinical setting and are seen as equally important to care as more task-oriented skills. It may be that Cox's ideas of structure are easier to apply where interpersonal skills are a key part of the therapeutic care being delivered.

Egan's three-stage model

Cox's three dimensions form 'structural boundaries' around the therapeutic interaction indicating what the practitioner uses to define the relationship. Egan's three-stage model could be considered as a model of the 'process' of a therapeutic interaction; defining the stages of the relationship.

Egan (1986) suggests three stages to the process of counselling, which are also applicable to any practitioner–patient relationship (Figure 7.1).

The first stage is identification of the problem. This may involve defining the problem or indeed exploring the key aspects of the problem. This stage is often about allowing the person to tell the story. The second stage is identifying and developing goals with the patient. This involves focusing on the problem and discovering the barriers to its solution. The third stage is about making plans that aim to achieve the goals. Often, this involves finding new ways of looking at the problem.

This whole process sounds very much like the first half of the nursing process of assessment, planning, implementation and evaluation. Indeed, it follows the same principles, but, critically, it is based on the patient's or client's values. Egan states that the

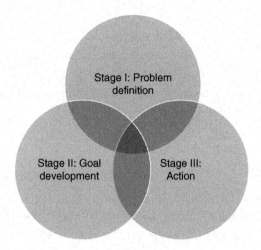

Figure 7.1 Egan's model of effective helping: overview (Egan 1986)

model is developmental and cumulative in that the success of each stage depends on the effectiveness of the previous stage. Let's look at Practice example box 7.1.

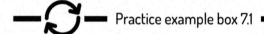 Practice example box 7.1

Egan's stages of helping

Jane is a 16-year-old with Down's syndrome. She is offered a place at residential college but her parents are worried that she will not cope away from home. Jane feels uneasy because she wants to go, but doesn't want to leave her parents. Her key worker helps Jane discuss the issues involved around coping and identifying what she is afraid of specifically. They decide that Jane is afraid of upsetting her parents by saying she wants to go to college. Jane and the key worker identify that Jane needs to communicate her desire to go and that her parents need to come to terms with her leaving home. They decide to have a focused family get-together with the key worker and the education advisor to discuss how everyone is feeling and allow everyone to air their concerns.

In the above example, we can see how Egan's model helps map the three stages of the helping process:

Stage I: The key worker and Jane identify the specific reason for Jane's anxieties.

Stage II: Jane and the key worker focus on the problem and identify the goals.

Stage III: They devise a plan to discuss the problem with the relevant people.

Egan's model is person-centred in that the problem identification and goals must be the patient's own ideas, and patient self-responsibility is key. The helper facilitates the person's problem-solving by guiding the problem-solving process but not advising, or making suggestions or decisions on behalf of the patient. The model is also circular and overlapping as stages need to be revisited to tackle each problem that arises.

Summary of humanistic approaches

With both Cox's and Egan's approaches to therapeutic interactions, the humanistic principles as adopted by Carl Rogers can be seen to apply. Both regard the client as taking responsibility for problem-solving and being able to respond to empowerment by engaging in the problem-solving process. It is the patient who has the answers, but the nurse who facilitates their discovery.

It could be argued, however, that humanistic principles are impossible to achieve while there is a power difference between the nurse and the patient. Rogers (1961) was proposing a mutual relationship in a counselling setting in which the client seeks and uses the therapist in a form of self-healing. In healthcare professions concerned with public health in general, the agenda may be to change the unhealthy behaviour of populations and individuals and to deliver health promotion. Arguably, some aspects of healthcare go beyond the developmental needs of the individual patient to population-based conformity with contemporary cultural health values; for instance, in forensic nursing an environment such as a prison or mental hospital essentially challenges the notion of person-centred freedom of choice (Jacob et al., 2008). A key theorist, Furedi (2002), maintains that we currently live in a risk-averse society that sets an agenda of protection and prevention. A health example of this may be expectations of compliance with treatment, with health screening and the promotion of healthy eating and smoking cessation.

Arguably, illness prevention and health promotion in nursing aim to change behaviour and make the assumption that they will be 'good' for the patient. The next section will look at a different approach to communication, aimed at behaviour change.

Behaviour change and communication

Behavioural explanations of human existence maintain that people learn what is good and useful in the environment and what is not good, not useful or, indeed, harmful by interacting with it. Socially, this means interacting with other people and striving to get on with others, and learning what to avoid. So, we learn as we develop socially and intellectually how to behave, think about and understand our environment in ways that are 'adaptive' – that is, advantageous – and avoid doing things we have learned are maladaptive – or disadvantageous.

As small children we soon learn that hitting our younger sister is disadvantageous because we get told off. However, we also learn that picking on our younger sister is fun (advantageous) if we can get away with it. So, we learn some very complex ways of behaving in our society as we grow up, and continue to learn how to adapt to new people, environments and situations like ill health through the principles of behavioural learning theory. The theory is often divided up into some key components, which we will examine.

Conditioning and reinforcement

When an animal, including a human, is exposed to an element in the environment for the first time, if something good happens at the same time, the animal associates that element with being good.

You have probably learned about Pavlov's experiment with dogs, in which the dogs heard a bell ringing every time they were fed. They soon anticipated food by salivating when they heard the bell, even when no food was present. A child will associate the chime of an ice cream van with a pleasant experience if they usually get an ice cream. Alternatively, a child may associate raised voices with fear of violence if they live in a violent household.

This type of **conditioning** is called **classical conditioning** because it conditions someone biologically to expect a rewarding or punishing experience when an environmental trigger is present.

What humans and animals can also do is change their behaviour when faced with certain environmental factors. This could be to gain a rewarding experience or avoid a punishing one. This ability to learn to control events is called **operant conditioning** and was identified by a behaviourist called Skinner who trained rats to operate a lever in a cage to get a food pellet (Skinner, 1973).

Suppose a child who lives in a violent household associates raised voices with being hit, or seeing someone they love being upset. By hiding or distracting themselves the child does not get hit or see the violence. The next time the shouting starts, the child is likely to use that strategy again because it avoids the painful experience. The child's avoidance behaviour is reinforced by a kind of reward – not having to experience as much of the trauma.

However, at school, this child may like the attention of a particular teacher, but the class is very big and the child doesn't stand out much. One day, the child is particularly frustrated and feeling bad and unloved, and hits another child. The child then gets lots of attention from the teacher. The next day, feeling bad, the child hits another classmate. This hitting behaviour has become a way of attracting attention and getting a positive stroke (see Chapter 3). Even being told off, for this child, is better than being ignored or being invisible.

The child's behaviour is 'reinforced' by the attention the child gets from the teacher. **Reinforcement** of behaviour requires a short-term association between the reinforcing stimuli and the 'pay off' because it is learned unconsciously. Humans can overcome this by learning consciously that longer-term consequences can be beneficial. For instance, most people would avoid the dentist but we are aware that the short-term discomfort is worth it in the long term. This is an important factor when it comes to overcoming unconscious learning. We will look at this in the next section, but first a quick reminder.

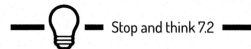 Stop and think 7.2

Can you think of stimuli you have become conditioned to that make you either feel nervous or happy? What about something you do to avoid something unpleasant? Remember:

Conditioning is associating one trigger with a particular experience, whether positive or negative.

Reinforcement is a positive environmental effect that is a consequence of behaviour. It takes the form either of a reward or avoidance of something unpleasant.

Use of classical conditioning can be incorporated into specialist approaches to change serious maladaptive behaviour such as drug or alcohol addiction, and inappropriate sexual behaviour, but is probably most commonly used in nursing for child bed-wetting, using an alarmed mattress that helps the child associate the feelings of a full bladder with waking up.

Operant conditioning is often called behaviour modification and, apart from being used in specialist psychology, can be used effectively by nurses to target health behaviour change such as smoking cessation (Roberts et al., 2013), wandering behaviour among people with dementia (Lai and Arthur, 2003) and obesity (Teixeira and Marques, 2017).

So, what has this to do with health communication? As health professionals we are often faced with patients, relatives and even colleagues who have learned maladaptive ways of behaving and thinking which prevents them from adopting healthy lifestyles or having healthy relations with others. Let's look at some case study examples in Box 7.2.

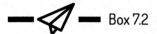 Box 7.2

Case studies of maladaptive behaviour

1   A middle-aged divorced man with no current employment feels low, lonely and worthless. He often drinks heavily to cheer himself up. This works in the short term so every time he feels

stressed, upset or depressed he drinks heavily. He has become alcohol-dependent, has liver damage, can't get a job because he is an alcoholic and his teenage children don't visit him anymore.

2 A teenage girl used to be teased at school because she was fat. She went on a diet and received lots of praise and attention for being slim. She now weighs 35 kg and is seriously underweight for her age and build.

3 An older man with treatable bowel cancer refuses to go to hospital for an operation because he believes he will die on the operating table. Two years ago, his wife had a simple operation and died in hospital.

4 A boy with severe autism won't go to school without wearing his Spiderman costume as he associates it with being protected from other people. Without it, he has severe temper tantrums and anxiety so his parents give in and let him wear his costume.

These examples are not uncommon patient problems. However, everyone we meet is subject to behavioural learning in some way, including ourselves. By understanding the principles of learning theory, we can incorporate them in our communication in professional relationships and guide people to more adaptive ways of engaging with health behaviour. Suggested answers to the problems posed in the case studies in Box 7.2 are outlined in Stop and think 7.3.

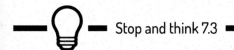 Stop and think 7.3

Before you read the suggested answers to the problems posed in the case studies in Box 7.2, take a minute to try to identify the likely conditioning triggers for the people in the case studies, and what reinforcement they are getting for their unhelpful behaviour.

Suggested answers:

1 The man is conditioned to associate alcohol with pleasure. His drinking behaviour is reinforced by avoiding negative feelings of stress and low mood by drinking. The more often he drinks, the more often he avoids feeling really bad and therefore the more often he will use alcohol to avoid negative feelings.

2 The teenage girl is conditioned to associate being fat with being rejected by others. She has learned that dieting/not eating avoids rejection and gains positive approval from others. Unfortunately, she has probably also associated not eating and feeling hungry with a sense of power over her body and other people and gets pleasure from resisting food.

3 The man has probably learned to associate the trauma of his wife's unexpected death with very powerful feelings of grief, shock and possibly fear and mistrust. He is conditioned to link hospitals with fear of death and loss. By resisting invitations to go into hospital for treatment, he feels a sense of relief from his fear. He is using avoidance behaviour to reduce his grief and fear of death.

(Continued)

4   A severely autistic child usually finds other people and unfamiliar surroundings very threatening. This boy has associated Spiderman (and probably his own identification with Spiderman) with safety and protection. The more he wears his costume, the more he will associate
safety with wearing it. He is also learning something else, which is maladaptive: his parents
give in when he has a temper tantrum, thus reinforcing his behaviour every time he gets his
own way.

The nurse–patient relationship has the potential to help service users learn more
positive ways of behaving and understanding situations through conditioning and reinforcement. The nurse can easily reward adaptive behaviour by communicating praise
and positive attention, and help reduce maladaptive behaviour with disapproval or lack
of response (no reward). All this is performed through communication. Let's look at
some examples.

Example 1: Avoiding reinforcement of maladaptive behaviour

A depressed woman often makes herself feel worse by talking about how awful she feels.
The nurse uses reinforcement to encourage the woman to talk positively and not dwell
on her troubles.

Nurse:	'Hello, how are you feeling today?'
Patient:	'Oh, nurse, I'm not good at all. I had those dreadful dreams in the night and woke up feeling worse than yesterday. I don't think I'll ever get better again.'
Nurse (not responding to the negative comments):	'What are you planning today that will lift your mood?'
Patient:	'I don't know. I can't think of anything.'
Nurse:	'You liked the art group yesterday. What did you think was good about it?'
Patient:	'Well, it took my mind off things for a while.'
Nurse:	'Good. That sounds like a great idea for today.'

The nurse deliberately avoids rewarding the negative comments by ignoring them.
Instead, the nurse encourages a positive comment and gives the patient a rewarding positive stroke when she says something less negative, and the nurse adds a suggestion that it
was the patient's idea.

Example 2: Teaching maladaptive behaviour and punishing adaptive behaviour

Conditioning can also be a very powerful factor in teaching maladaptive behaviour through inappropriate reinforcement. The power imbalance in the nurse–patient relationship can have a negative effect on people by reinforcing maladaptive behaviour. A good example of this is institutionalisation whereby long-term patients such as those in care for older people, mental health rehabilitation or learning disability homes can become very dependent and compliant if overly controlled by the social environment (Goffman, 1961).

In hospital a very reluctant child finally agrees to take his medication. The nurse has been getting frustrated by the child's previous refusals and replies:

Nurse: 'So I should think, after all that fuss!'

Here, the nurse has not rewarded the child for the adaptive behaviour, but made the child feel guilty (given punishment) for not complying in the first place. This child is unlikely to comply any more readily next time.

Example 3: Rewarding maladaptive behaviour

A patient in a psychiatric ward has deliberately cut her arm while feeling very upset and distressed. She shows the nurse the wound, who says:

Nurse: 'Oh your poor thing! You must have been feeling awful to do this. Let me stitch that up for you. What made you do this? I can't imagine what you must have been feeling to do this to yourself!'

The patient needs attention but not the sort that will encourage more self-harming behaviour. The nurse could attend to the wound but talk about something else that is not rewarding. What she needs to avoid is both punishing the patient by telling her off and rewarding her by giving undue attention. The nurse could focus on what the patient could do instead of self-harming, such as talking to someone about how she feels, and encourage that behaviour instead with praise and positive attention.

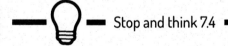 Stop and think 7.4

Reflect on a situation you may have encountered in practice or in another aspect of your life where you met someone who seemed to be seeking your attention and you couldn't get away. This may have been a patient who wanted to talk or a child who wanted to keep showing you

(Continued)

their toys. Considering the material above about rewarding through attention, what do you think were the factors that made this person persist in gaining your attention? What were you doing to reward this behaviour? What could you have done instead? Look ahead to Chapter 8 and the section on Being assertive and saying 'no' for clues! You should also reflect on such incidents when they occur in practice and consider how you have used rewarding or non-rewarding behaviour to control the encounter.

Social learning theory

Modelling

It is not just by through experiencing the environment directly that we learn what is rewarding or unpleasant. Another way we learn about ourselves is through watching other people. Thus the nurse can become a role model for what is possible, or guide the person to other role models, reducing fear or anxiety and developing adaptive behaviour.

Have you ever watched a frightening film and been scared just because the characters in the film are scared? Why do you think you are scared? You are safe at home and there are no monsters or murderers lurking in the cupboards. You have 'identified' with the characters in the film and are experiencing their environment vicariously (through their eyes). Alternatively, have you ever done something challenging because you have seen someone else do it successfully? This is the principle of **vicarious learning** (Bandura, 1977); learning by observing others. People who have phobias about spiders, for example, may undergo exposure therapy. This may involve watching the therapist handle a spider before they handle the spider themselves.

The important element to this kind of learning is the relationship between the watcher and the person performing the behaviour. If the watcher cannot identify with the performer, they will not experience vicarious learning. You might watch a daredevil motorcyclist successfully leap a row of buses, but you probably would not identify with them and want have a go yourself.

The autistic boy in Stop and think 7.3 associated safety with becoming Spiderman through watching a film. He learned this vicariously, and this conditioning was reinforced by not coming to harm when wearing his costume. Let's see some further examples.

Example 4: Identification and role modelling

A 5-year-old child at a diabetes clinic is learning to have insulin injections. The nurse tells a story about how the teddy at the clinic has insulin injections but he doesn't mind. The nurse shows the child how the teddy has his insulin and how teddy can then go and play.

The nurse has communicated to the child that having an insulin injection is routine and allows people to lead a normal life. The nurse is using role modelling through the teddy and the child is learning vicariously by identifying with the teddy.

Example 5: Role modelling unprofessional behaviour

An annoyed staff nurse walks into the office in which a student nurse and two health-care assistants are sitting. She says:

Nurse: 'That doctor is so lazy! I've had to do all the bloods and observations for him while he just watched and ordered me about. He likes to show off in front of the patients! He doesn't know anything about teamwork!'

This nurse, while obviously annoyed, has modelled unprofessional behaviour in front of junior staff by denigrating a member of the multi-disciplinary team. The junior staff members are likely to copy this behaviour – even if it includes denigrating the staff nurse!

Self-efficacy

The last important element to learning theory that we will cover is **self-efficacy**. Self-efficacy is the innate concept of ourselves that, whatever happens, we have the ability to do something positive, believe that we will survive and have the confidence to rely on our own inner resources to get through. Albert Bandura described self-efficacy as the belief that one can perform effectively, and this is brought about best by actually overcoming feared or difficult situations (Bandura, 1977).

If you do something you never thought you'd be able to do, you are likely to experience a great sense of wellbeing, pride and good self-esteem. If you perceive it as a major achievement, you are likely to go on to do other things you previously thought were beyond your capabilities. Young people from deprived backgrounds who go on outward bound courses and conquer mountains, a non-runner who completes a marathon and students with learning disabilities who gain a degree: all are examples of people whose confidence is boosted by their achievements because their sense of self-efficacy has increased massively.

Nurses have the opportunity to develop another's self-efficacy by changing the way they see themselves and what they think they are capable of. For example, Lee et al. (2008) found improved and maintained exercise activity among older people when the theory of self-efficacy was incorporated into exercise programmes. These programmes included using verbal encouragement and helping people feel good about their exercise (rewarding), vicarious learning (watching others achieve) and the experience of achievement (self-efficacy).

However, nurses are also in a position to reduce someone's self-efficacy by encouraging dependence.

Example 6: Encouraging dependency and reducing self-efficacy

A nurse is with the anxious parent of a young boy with cerebral palsy. He has tantrums and becomes aggressive when he can't do things his brothers can do. His mother is very stressed.

Mother: 'I can't cope when he has a tantrum. He's too big for me to manage now. I don't know what's going to happen in the future. I won't be able to cope'.

Nurse: 'It is very hard. That's why you need lots of support. I and my colleagues will always be able to give advice and support when you need it'.

Apart from promising support in the future that may not be there, the nurse is reinforcing the thought that the parent won't be able to cope on her own. This takes away the sense of self-efficacy the mother needs to build up.

The nurse could have said:

Nurse: 'You might not think so now, but you will discover ways of coping. What we could do now is explore those together and help you find solutions'.

This does not reinforce a sense of dependency but encourages the person to be realistic but hopeful. It does promise collaboration, which is realistic, and better coping in the future.

Summary of behavioural approaches

Behavioural approaches to human relations could be seen as incompatible with the humanistic philosophy. In some ways they empower the practitioner to manipulate the patient into behaviour change. The result can often be that not only does the person behave in a different way, but they may not realise that they have been unconsciously guided into changing their behaviour.

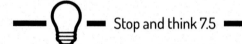 Stop and think 7.5

How do you think nurses can justify using a behavioural approach to changing a person's lifestyle while still adhering to the person-centred philosophy?

Possible answer: this is a critical debate about how healthcare is provided, from the level of international government down to the level of the nurse–patient relationship. We can question to what extent healthcare is benevolent and whether it can be too controlling and interfere in people's lives. The nurse can, however, determine what the patient ultimately wants, and use a behavioural approach to help them achieve it. An expressed desire to lose weight, stop using drugs or gain better anger management can all be aided by behavioural modification approaches. The nurse always needs to be mindful, however, that this is what the patient wants and their human rights are not violated.

It may also be as important for nurses to understand how their power can affect a patient's behaviour, and avoid reinforcing maladaptive behaviour or discouraging adaptive behaviour.

The cognitive behavioural approach

An approach that is expanding from its original mental health roots into other health settings is **cognitive behavioural therapy** (CBT). It is described as a talking therapy (NHS UK, 2017). It is the recommended therapeutic approach for depression and anxiety-related psychiatric problems, and for interventions for schizophrenia symptom control (NICE, 2019). However, it has expanded across a range of healthcare fields as a health promotion approach, for example in type 2 diabetes (De Groot et al., 2016), and can be delivered effectively by nurses (Heslop et al., 2009; Warrilow and Beech, 2009; Currid et al., 2011). Possibly an important element to the development of CBT is that it empowers the individual patient to make choices and change behaviour, and therefore may have a stronger claim to being an ethically based practice than the purely behavioural approach.

CBT was first described as the 'cognitive triad' (Beck, 1976) because it addresses behaviour, cognition and physical/emotional responses, and recognises that these elements are dynamically linked. The principles of CBT are the same as behavioural and social learning theory but, instead of focusing on what people do, it focuses on how people think about and perceive their situation. It recognises that people are conditioned to associate one thing with another, but also that we often learn how to think about situations in ways that are maladaptive, just because they may have worked once or in the short term.

Figure 7.2 illustrates the sequence of events using the three systems of thoughts, feelings and behaviour that link how we perceive a situation and consequently respond.

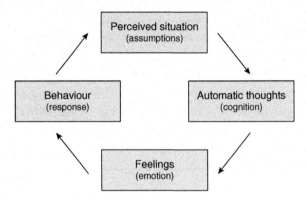

Figure 7.2 The three system cycle and its links to perception

A maladaptive sequence of events may be as shown in Box 7.3.

 Box 7.3

A maladaptive cycle of fear

A needle-phobic patient is about to have a blood sample taken.

Perceived situation: this is a bad situation for me.

Automatic thoughts: I will have a panic attack, lose control, look stupid and not cope. People will think I'm a coward, a baby or mad if I panic and have to run out of here.

Feelings: mounting anxiety, fear, panic and experiencing a need to escape, feeling trapped and being out of control. Physical symptoms of panic (feeling sick, wobbly, high blood pressure, pulse and respiration rates, sweating and tingling).

Behaviour: looking for escape routes, asking if it really needs to be done, wanting to leave, not allowing the nurse to perform the procedure.

Perceived situation: interpretation of having a blood test confirmed (reinforced) by the negative experience: 'I thought this would be bad, and it is.'

We will add a good nursing intervention to this scenario. The nurse understands the cycle of panic that links thoughts to feelings and behaviour and notices that the patient looks worried. The nurse could use several different ways to interrupt this patient's cycle of maladaptive thinking, feeling and behaving.

1   If the anxiety is mild:
    • change the thoughts from negative to positive: remind the patient that it will help resolve their health problems when the results are back.

2   If the anxiety is more marked:

- distract the patient from thinking about what is happening: ask about their journey to the hospital, what they may be doing later, where they bought that lovely jacket from – anything that makes the patient focus on something rewarding about themselves rather than their fear.

3   If the anxiety is serious:

- put the patient in control: ask what would help the patient have the procedure done less traumatically. Do they want to say when to do it, do they want the door open or closed and do they need privacy (to combat the 'everyone will think I'm stupid' thoughts)? Reassure the patient that other people hate needles and so it's not a stupid thing to worry about.

Many of us would perform these reassuring communications automatically to help a worried patient, but by understanding what may be happening for the patient the nurse can easily assess the patient's perceptions and thoughts, and judge which communication intervention is most appropriate.

In the example above, certain automatic thoughts may seem absurd or irrational. However, we may have developed habitual use of certain ways of thinking. They epitomise how we see the world and interpret our role in it. In CBT, these 'unhelpful' or 'maladaptive' thoughts are regarded as dysfunctional because they stop us thinking about a situation realistically.

Dysfunctional thinking styles

Dysfunctional thinking has been defined in a classic CBT text as being:

> beliefs which individuals hold about the world and themselves which [...]
> make them prone to interpret specific situations in an excessively negative and
> dysfunctional fashion.

> (Hawton et al., 1989:55)

Certain words or phrases people use indicate to the listener how they perceive themselves and the world. Nurses listening attentively can pick up on negative statements that are not realistic and challenge the patient to revise their way of thinking. See Table 7.1 for some examples of dysfunctional negative thinking and the kind of phrases that give clues to the patient's assumptions.

There's nothing wrong with recognising the reality of a situation, but, if the person is making an assumption, we can challenge their view of the world. The key to detecting unhelpful thinking is whether it is *realistic*. If the statement suggests the person has a realistic understanding of the situation, this indicates helpful thinking. See Table 7.2 for some very common examples of unhelpful thinking in healthcare.

Table 7.1   Examples of dysfunctional thinking

Common negative unrealistic thoughts (examples)	Realistic alternative (negative)	Realistic alternative (positive)
I can't ... learn to inject myself.	I might not be able to.	I might be able to.
It's not fair ... that I have this disease.	My life will change for the worse.	I don't know how my life will change.
I will fail/look stupid ... by attending group therapy.	I am afraid to try in case I don't fit in.	I might fit in if I try. But it doesn't matter if I don't (what's the worst that could happen?).
They won't like me ... at the day centre.	I am afraid to go in case I don't like it.	It doesn't matter if I don't like it, I can still go and see.

Table 7.2   Examples of unhelpful thinking

Unhelpful word	Example	Reasons why word is unhelpful
can't	'I *can't* stop smoking.'	Restricts options and doesn't look at the evidence.
should	'I *should* be able to remember... .'	Why? Imposes too great an expectation on self and sets the person up to experience failure.
shouldn't	'She *shouldn't* talk to me like that.'	But she does! That's the reality. Leads to unhelpful thoughts such as 'it's not fair'.
must	'I *must* do better at ... .'	Who says? This makes an outcome dependent on certain behaviour. Sets the person up to fail.
wouldn't	'I *wouldn't* have to do this if ... .' (This is very common among nursing teams!)	How do you know? The reality is that the person *has chosen* to do this. There is always a choice.
ought	'I *ought* to know better.'	Not recognising the reality and setting unachievable standards; expectations are too high.

Useful challenges to unrealistic thinking feature words and phrases such as: Why? Who says? Where's your evidence? How do you know? See Practice example box 7.2.

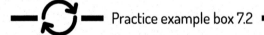 Practice example box 7.2

Challenging negative thoughts

A patient insisted she couldn't go on a beach holiday because her burn scars looked so horrible. She said she would feel that everyone was looking at her and thinking she *should* cover herself up in public. The nurse picked up on her assumptions about what people would think and identified that 'should' meant people would judge her by her appearance. The nurse and patient examined the assumptions behind her thoughts and concluded that people would be unlikely to judge her negatively or think badly of her, and that anyway it did not matter as it was their problem, not hers.

The woman went on the beach holiday.

Whenever you find yourself with a patient who appears 'stuck' in a form of unhealthy behaviour or not complying with treatment, listen to the reasons the person gives for their behaviour. You may pick up on phrases or words used that suggest the person's unhealthy thinking style which may lie at the root of their problems in changing behaviour.

....

Knowledge link You will find an example of humanistic and behavioural models working together in Chapter 15 on motivational interviewing.

....

Conclusion

This chapter links to previous chapters in Part 1 on the nurse–patient relationship and active listening, and further chapters in Part 3, particularly on promoting health. The earlier chapters outline the basic skills and theories of communication and this chapter illustrates some of the models or approaches which provide a framework for those skills. Part 3 will address both the basic skills and the frameworks in application to specific health-related practice.

....FURTHER READING

Kennerley, H., Kirk, J. and Westbrook, D. (2017) *An Introduction to Cognitive Behaviour Therapy: Skills and Applications* (3rd edn). London, SAGE Publications.

....REFERENCES

Adams, L. (2016) The conundrum of caring in nursing. *International Journal of Caring Sciences*, 9(1), 1–8.

Bandura, A. (1977) *Social Learning Theory*. Englewood Cliffs, NJ, Prentice Hall.

Beck, A. (1976) *Cognitive Therapy and the Emotional Disorders*. New York, International Universities Press.

Cox, M. (1978) *Structuring the Therapeutic Process: Compromise with Chaos*. London, Jessica Kingsley Press.

Currid, T.J., Nikcĕvic, A. and Spada, M.M. (2011) Cognitive behavioural therapy and its relevance to nursing. *British Journal of Nursing*, 20(11), 1443–1447.

de Groot, M., Golden, S.H. and Wagner, J. (2016) Psychological conditions in adults with diabetes. *The American Psychologist*, 71(7), 552–562.

Egan, G. (1986) *The Skilled Helper: A Systematic Approach to Effective Helping*. Belmont, CA, Brooks/Cole.

Furedi, F. (2002) *The Culture of Fear: Risk-taking and the Morality of Low Expectation Risk-taking*. London, Continuum.

Goffman, E. (1961) *Asylums*. Harmondsworth, Penguin Books.

Hawton, K., Salkovskis, P.M., Kirk, J. and Clark, D.M. (1989) *Cognitive Behaviour Therapy for Psychiatric Problems: A Practical Guide*. Oxford, Oxford Medical Publications.

Heslop, K., De Soya, A., Baker, C., Stenton, C. and Burns, G. (2009) Using individualised cognitive behavioural therapy as a treatment for people with COPD. *Nursing Times*, 105(14), 14–17.

Jacob, J., Holmes, D. and Buus, N. (2008) Humanism in forensic psychiatry: the use of the tidal nursing model. *Nursing Inquiry*, 15(3), 224–230.

Lai, C. and Arthur, D. (2003) Wandering behaviour in people with dementia. *Journal of Advanced Nursing*, 44(2), 173–182.

Lee, L.-L., Antony, A. and Avis, M. (2008) Using self-efficacy theory to develop interventions that help older people overcome psychological barriers to physical activity. *International Journal of Nursing Studies*, 45(11), 1690–1699.

Maslow, A. (1970) *Motivation and Personality*. New York, Harper & Row.

NHS UK (2017) *Overview; Cognitive Behavioural Therapy (CBT)*. www.nhs.uk/conditions/cognitive-behavioural-therapy-cbt/.

NICE (2019) *Cognitive Behaviour Therapy for Psychosis can be Adapted and Implemented for Minority Ethnic Groups: a Randomised Controlled Trial*. www.nice.org.uk/sharedlearning/cognitive-behaviour-therapy-for-psychosis-can-be-adapted-and-implemented-for-minority-ethnic-groups-a-randomised-controlled-trial.

NMC (2018) *The Code: Professional Standards of Practice and Behaviour for Nurses, Midwives and Nursing Associates*. www.nmc.org.uk/standards/code/.

Roberts, N.J., Kerr, S.M. and Smith, S.M. (2013) Behavioral interventions associated with smoking cessation in the treatment of tobacco use. *Health Services Insights*, 6, 79–85.

Rogers, C. (1961) *On Becoming a Person: A Therapist's View of Psychotherapy*. London, Constable.

Skinner, B. (1973) *Beyond Freedom & Dignity*. Penguin, Harmsworth.

Teixeira, P.J. and Marques, M.M. (2017) Health behavior change for obesity management. *Obesity Facts*, 10, 666–673.

Warrilow, A. and Beech, B. (2009) Self-help CBT for depression: opportunities for primary care mental health nurses? *Journal of Psychiatric and Mental Health Nursing*, 16(9), 792–803.

EIGHT
FACING CHALLENGES IN HEALTHCARE COMMUNICATION
LUCY WEBB AND CLEMENTINAH ROOKE

.... THIS CHAPTER WILL HELP YOU TO:

- Recognise and overcome barriers to developing effective relationships with patients
- Be accepting of different cultural traditions, beliefs, UK legal frameworks and professional ethics
- Manage and diffuse challenging situations
- Make appropriate use of the environment, self and skills
- Communicate sensitively in different settings, using a range of methods and skills
- Select and apply appropriate strategies and techniques for conflict resolution, de-escalation and physical intervention in the management of potential violence and aggression

Introduction

This chapter outlines some of the hazards and challenges often met when attempting communication in a range of health settings. We will give tips, advice and guidance on common difficulties found in challenging circumstances such as in the patient's home, when there is a cultural difference or a language difference, when professional boundaries are crossed or when others are hostile or unwilling. This will also include development of skills to help the student manage communication that they personally find difficult.

The home visit

Community nurses often deliver care in the patient's own home. This can present several communication challenges from the outset, even before tackling the health need itself. As you have seen in Chapter 1, communication can be seen in light of power dynamics, where power is often enhanced for the nurse because the patient is out of their comfort zone, while the nurse is surrounded by supportive colleagues and the trappings of power such as a uniform and institutionalised processes and customs.

Common problems

When we visit a patient in their own home the balance of power shifts towards the patient. The nurse becomes subject to the rules and social customs of being a guest in someone else's house. We will need to be invited inside, may be required to take our shoes off when entering, will need to ask to use resources such as a basin, toilet or rubbish bin, and may have to negotiate around offers of tea and coffee. As a health professional in the community, we may be on our own or be a student with a lone practitioner, while our patient may have family and friends present. Also, the environment itself can present factors we have little control over. Children love to be involved with whatever is going on and often seek attention. Pets can be similarly distracting. We rely on the patient or relative to control these distractions. People may have visitors when we call, or phone calls from chatty friends. Many people keep their televisions switched on when a visitor arrives. This is distracting for both the patient and the nurse and presents a communication barrier.

To get the best out of your nurse–patient interaction in the patient's home, you need to ensure the environment is suitable for good communication. You may need to be assertive and take charge, while being sensitive to issues of consent.

Being assertive

Many people being visited at home by a health professional will view that person as an authority figure with skills they depend on. They will be quite happy for you to set the agenda for your visit, to be business-like and to take charge. By being assertive from the outset, you are not likely to present the patient with anything unexpected. Assertiveness is a personal skill or quality that enables a person to give their opinions and manage their social boundaries without aggressiveness or passive submission. An assertive person can give instructions and say 'no' to others in a way that demonstrates confidence and flexibility. So, how do we use assertiveness to control the environment in a patient's home?

Set the boundaries for the encounter at the outset

Here's an example:

> 'Hello. Are you Mrs Smith? I am [your full name], the student nurse from the surgery. I've come to check your dressings. It should only take about 10 minutes. Is now a good time?'

This is a good opening. You have stated your intent, your time boundary and your task boundary (what you are visiting for). You have also given the person an opportunity to give consent. After all, it might be a very difficult time for Mrs Smith: the boiler may have just broken down!

When inside, check the environment for anything that might present a communication barrier, especially if you are likely to have an exchange that requires privacy and sensitivity.

Which room is best to use? Mrs Smith is about to lead you to the kitchen where you can see Mr Smith having his lunch. You can see the living room is free.

> 'Shall we go in here, Mrs Smith? There's probably more room, and I don't want to disturb Mr Smith.'

By simply directing Mrs Smith politely to what *you* want, you have asserted that your judgement is important. But you have given her the choice; after all, it is her home.

The television is on and quite loud as Mrs Smith is hard of hearing.

> 'I'll just turn the television off, so we can talk properly.'

Turn off the television rather than turning the sound down, as pictures are distracting too.

Mr Smith wanders in when he's finished his lunch and takes an interest in what you are doing. You will have to judge if this is a problem for Mrs Smith as it could constitute a breach of confidentiality or more simply interfere with any intimate issues she might want to discuss with you. It may be up to you to protect the privacy and dignity of your patient. The nurse may be required to take charge of the situation and exclude Mr Smith, but asking someone to leave their own living room is ethically tricky. In this situation, it is appropriate to use the authority of the health professional but you still need to elicit co-operation and consent.

> 'Mr Smith, I just need to see Mrs Smith alone for a few moments while I do my assessment. Would you mind waiting outside until I have finished?'

Note the use of *I*, as in you, the nurse/health professional/expert, and not *we*, as in you and Mrs Smith. This asserts that you, the professional, have a job to do and you are required to do it in a certain way. It does not compromise the relationship between Mr and Mrs Smith.

Saying 'no' assertively

In many home situations the health professional is more likely to be overwhelmed with kindness rather than need to direct others. This sort of scenario also requires assertiveness, because a community worker can only drink so many cups of tea a day and needs to get all their appointments done on time! So, assertiveness is important in limiting the amount of time and attention you can give. Start as you mean to go on by setting your boundaries.

> 'This will only take 10 minutes.'

This is a good time as it makes clear the time you have got to spare.

> 'No tea today, thank you. I've got quite a bit to do today. Now, let's have a look at that leg and you can tell me how you are getting on.'

In other words, you can't stop for long and need to get down to business, but you still have time to listen to the patient's difficulties.

There are lots of ways to say 'no', but not all of them are assertive. Look at the list in Box 8.1 and see which you think are assertive and which are non-assertive (passive).

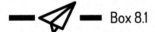 **Box 8.1**

Assertive and non-assertive statements

- No, thank you.
- I'd rather not.
- No, I'm fine thanks.
- I don't think that's a good idea.
- No, not that way.
- That's not quite right.
- No.

Easy, isn't it? All the assertive phrases have the word 'no' in them. We don't like to hurt people's feelings, but 'no' is the easiest way to say 'no'. Most phrases of refusal that do not contain the word 'no' are not as assertive as ones that do.

And, when pressed, simply repeat the word – in another way, if you like (see Box 8.2).

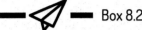 **Box 8.2**

Reinforcing assertiveness

- No, honestly, I can't.
- No, really.

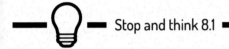 **Stop and think 8.1**

Next time you want to refuse something, note how you phrase it. Are you good at saying 'no'? When are you not good at saying 'no'? In what circumstances, with whom and where?

Cultural difference and using interpreters

Whole books have been written on culture and cultural differences in healthcare so this part of the chapter aims to focus specifically on problem-solving in order to reduce the communication barriers presented by culture and language differences. Further reading is provided at the end of the chapter for those who would like to explore the subject in more detail for assignments (see also Chapter 6 in this book).

According to Houghton (2016), culture consists of knowledge, beliefs, behaviours, laws and customs, objects and other aspects common to members of a particular group of society such as language, values and norms, tools, technologies, products, organisations and institutions (family, religion, education and healthcare). However, he is quick to point out that the terms 'culture' and 'society' have lost some of their usefulness due to modern developments which have made it possible for people to interact and share resources globally. Arguably, the NMC (2018), in its latest proficiency standards for the 'future nurse', appears to acknowledge this loss of usefulness. The governing body places great emphasis on the need for a practitioner fully immersed in the global health agenda. It is therefore incumbent upon all nurses to have an appreciation of the dynamism of both culture and society and how this can impact on care delivery.

We are all influenced by our culture but often find it difficult to discern our own – which to us is 'normal' – unless we are faced with 'difference'. Also, we usually recognise the difference in communication 'rules' that suddenly present us with misunderstandings. The dilemma is more marked for immigrant nurses who have no choice but to navigate several cultures. Consider, for example, nurses from a culture which values spiritual healing as equally as medical interventions. Operating in a culture prohibiting the former would be an issue for them. Holland and Hogg (2010) warn that every nurse–patient relationship involves three cultures: those of the nurse, the patient and the organisation. As we identified earlier in this chapter, the nurse is likely to be more comfortable with the organisational culture, putting the patient in a doubly uncomfortable position in this relationship. In the case of the immigrant nurse or patient, the patient's dilemma is tripled.

The subtleties of meaning in interpersonal communication between two people of a similar culture or even sub-culture often come down to shared cultural phrases, facial expressions, gestures and even inflections (DeVito, 1988). You only have to observe two young teenagers conversing to realise that their 'culture' of age and role in society confers language and communication norms all of their own. Verbal expressions can mean one thing to one social culture and quite the opposite in another. For example, it took a while for the older generation to realise that a young person may use the word 'sick' to mean good! This could be very confusing unless the individuals on either side of the conversation make adjustments. The same could apply to gestures or inflections.

If we extrapolate from generational culture to ethnic differences, we can see that unless we all understand, recognise and make adjustments to different cultural meanings, communication between cultures will be full of misunderstanding and mis-communication. This should be a concern for nurses who are committed to ensuring social inclusion and respecting diversity and the beliefs, rights and wishes of individuals, groups and communities, and are expected to challenge inequality discrimination or exclusion from access to care (NMC, 2010). It is recognised that certain cultural and ethnic groups have particular healthcare needs and face specific barriers to healthcare. Asylum seekers and refugees may have specific health problems resulting from physical and mental trauma and often face social isolation, lack of understanding and barriers of language and communication (Burnett and Peel, 2001). For instance, people from these communities may lack access to information on health and not understand how to access healthcare (Kang et al., 2019). Women are less likely to speak English or be the spokesperson for the family in traditionally male-led cultures, and unaccompanied children are likely to be particularly vulnerable and need social care and support (Burnett and Peel, 2001). Let's have a look at some common problems.

Cultural difference

Clearly, the most obvious communication barriers are when two people do not understand the other's language. For some simple situations, and between people who at least share similar cultures, this may not be such a problem as gestures at least are similar between the two. For example, take two Western Europeans who share a general ethnic culture but not language. One could easily gesture a simple message such as 'I'm in pain' that would be quite clear to the other, and indicate where the pain is and how bad it is.

Two people of markedly different cultures and languages, however, may find this harder. For example, expressing pain may be socially unacceptable in the patient's culture, or pointing to signify 'you' or 'I' may simply confuse a patient who regards pointing as rude or aggressive. In Western medicine, health and illness are regarded as physical entities that are separate from spirituality or social wellbeing. However, in some health belief systems there is no division between the body and the mind or spirit and illness may be explained in terms of a person's poor moral behaviour or being possessed by something evil. Understanding of cultural expressions of health and illness requires us to take into account the values, norms and ways of understanding that the person has been brought up with. The person's health beliefs, whether patient or nurse, may include the individual's cultural definition of health, their environment (including the physical, social and symbolic environment they are and have been in) and cultural variations around their own health practices, beliefs, taboos and rites of passage (Holland and Hogg, 2010). These are simply the challenges nurses in modern society must contend with. See Practice example box 8.1 for a real practice example of a clash of symbolisms that stems from different values and experiences.

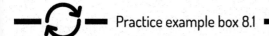 Practice example box 8.1

Differences in cultural symbolism

A young black gay man, a recent immigrant to the UK from a southern African country, was referred to a community mental health team in the UK with worrying symptoms of paranoia. In allocating a nurse key worker, it was agreed that a particular male nurse would be suitable because of the match in age and sex. However, the nurse was a white, rugby-playing, rather macho character while the patient had been brought up in a persecutory social environment in which homosexuality was illegal and highly stigmatised, and rugby was the cultural domain of the white ex-colonial population. It appeared that the referral decision had not addressed the different values of masculinity, homosexuality and social divisions between the patient and the nurse.

Expressions of culture in communication can also be different with respect to acceptable personal space, touch and making direct eye contact. The health professional's awareness of non-verbal expression is important as it can enhance the ability to deliver care. A case in point would be the experience of pain, which varies between communities due to the combination of language and cultural norms (Liao et al., 2016). People who are not used to the Western approach to medicine can be unused to the specific way in which pain is described or experienced. In a comparison between European mountain climbers and Nepalese mountain porters, for example, the porters would not report the European's pain experience as 'painful' perhaps because they regarded 'pain' simply as a normal experience (Halliday, 1992). Therefore, if a person with this belief system were asked 'where is the pain?' they may report that there is no pain.

In a ground-breaking study of women with cervical cancer, Bond and Pearson (1969) found that expressed pain varied depending on the women's personality type; the higher the woman's emotionality, the more painkillers she requested. The essential skills of communication that a health professional should possess is to remember that cultural issues should not be reduced to obvious 'expressions' of culture (and religion) such as dress, food or skin colour, but as an aspect of care which is unique to each individual patient, whatever their background.

Burnett and Peel (2001) suggest six key points, summarised here, that may help guide the health practitioner.

1 People have differing experiences and expectations of healthcare. They are not a homogeneous group.
2 Symptoms of psychological distress do not necessarily signify mental illness.
3 Trained interpreters or advocates should be used.
4 Community organisations can reduce isolation.
5 Particular difficulties faced by women can often be overlooked.
6 Support for children, especially if unaccompanied, needs to be multifaceted and multi-agency.

Language difference and the use of interpreters

Nurses in many open societies are likely to encounter people with very little linguistic and cultural understanding of the society they are in; for example, migrant workers and their families, asylum seekers and refugees. In such cases, it may be seen that having an interpreter would be the ideal solution where language difference is a communication barrier, but this in itself can present problems which it is helpful to be aware of. Box 8.3 illustrates a classic problem with using an interpreter.

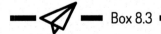 Box 8.3

The specialist sign language interpreter's perspective

'I try to remain simply an objective tool for interpretation but this is often impossible. A deaf patient with a psychotic illness kept asking me to help him as he didn't trust the nurse conducting the interview. I tried to reassure him but had to translate what I was saying for the nurse's benefit. If the nurse said anything to me, I needed to translate that as well to the deaf person. The patient wanted to see me as someone on his side and asked me not to translate everything he said. The nurse then got frustrated because he didn't know what we were saying. The nurse was unhelpful because he didn't recognise the difficulty I was having in remaining objective and kept including me in the conversation. In the end I had to tell both of them how to use me in the role effectively.'

It is difficult to have a third party present without that person becoming part of the triad rather than just facilitating a dyad.

....

Knowledge link See Chapter 5 for an introduction to dyads and triads.

....

Nurses are now required to recognise the need for an interpreter (NMC, 2010) to support communication. To do that, we need to understand how interpreters can facilitate or present a barrier to communication. Professional interpreters are trained to keep their role as objective as possible but also to help the two inter-locutors understand each other's position. The professional interpreter 'interprets' meanings rather than just translating (Tribe, 2007). A sign-language interpreter, for instance, may advise the hearing person about the pace of speech or gestures of the deaf person. A language interpreter may also advise people of any cultural misun-derstandings associated with expressions or behaviour. For example, close proximity may be quite uncomfortable for one and normal for the other. A good interpreter will be aware of this and give advice.

Unfortunately, professional and specialist interpreters are rarely available for routine and daily communication so healthcare workers often rely on health colleagues or fam-ily and friends of the patient (Hadziabdic et al., 2014). This presents many problems that a practitioner needs to be aware of, as outlined below.

1   Using an adult relative presents confidentiality problems and sometimes reluctance from the patient to divulge personal information. Also, a close relative often speaks *for* the patient rather than represent the patient's own communication accurately; i.e. 'my wife is fine, she doesn't want to make any fuss'.
2   Using children: often it is the case that children of first-generation immigrant families speak the host language better than the parents. This is a threat to confidentiality and there is also the possibility of parental inhibition as parents may feel uncomfortable in discussing health and social issues with their children present. Importantly, using a child to interpret could also be seen as exposing the child to harm. See Practice example box 8.2 for a real-life example.

3   Using other non-professional interpreters: again, there is a confidentiality issue if the interpreter is not a qualified health or social care professional. Also, non-professional interpreters have a tendency to get over-involved with the issues being discussed. Additionally, where small minority populations are concerned, often the informal interpreter has knowledge of the patient. See Practice example box 8.3 for a real example.

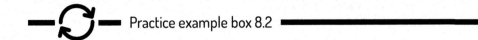 Practice example box 8.2

A child as an interpreter

A Tamil-speaking man arrived in a London hospital emergency department with delirium tremens. He was hallucinating, distressed and very frightened and suspicious. His wife and child (a boy of 10) accompanied him.

Emergency department staff and the mother initially relied on the boy to translate information about what was wrong and pass on reassurance from the staff to the mother and the father. The boy was therefore present and witnessed his father behaving in a distressed manner and had to translate details about his alcoholism, hallucinations and anxieties. He also had to pass on reassurance to his parents in a form of parent–child role reversal. Senior staff recognised that this situation was likely to put the child at emotional risk. The assessment was postponed until a Tamil-speaking doctor was found from another department to act as interpreter.

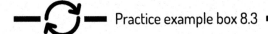 Practice example box 8.3

The informal interpreter

A Portuguese man needed to give informed consent to a fairly routine but personal treatment procedure. A professional interpreter was not available for many hours, potentially delaying the procedure. However, a hospital-wide search found a member of the catering staff who was Portuguese and spoke good English. This woman was pleased to help and translated the information the man needed, and he clearly consented to the procedure. On leaving the ward, the woman then said to the nurse as an aside that she knew his family, they were a bad sort and she wasn't surprised he had become ill!

Modern technology has brought with it recent developments in video and telephonic interpretation services closely resembling face-to-face interactions, thus allowing optimisation of scarce resources (Masland et al., 2010; Osae-Larbi, 2016). Their use is said to have increased because they are user-friendly, provide rapid access to interpretation and reduce waiting times (Masland et al., 2010).

Guidance for working with interpreters

From the above examples and evidence, we can find simple but worthwhile practices when dealing with language differences.

When using a professional interpreter:

1   Be aware of the need to remain a dyad between patient and nurse, with you as the facilitator, rather than allowing the conversation to become a triad. Watch your boundaries.
2   Check with your interpreter beforehand for any cultural rules or guidelines that the interpreter needs you to follow.
3   Ensure your interpreter remains professionally objective during the interview but recognise that sometimes it is useful, and fairly likely, if the patient experiences relief and assurance from having someone to talk to in their own language.

When using a non-professional interpreter:

1   Ensure confidentiality as much as possible – you can be guided by what is in the patient's best interests.
2   Check for any Trust or employer guidelines or policies on use of non-professional interpreters.
3   *Do not* use children as interpreters for anything except simple and routine communication. Therapeutic, diagnostic, placatory or other interventional communications are likely to place the child at risk of emotional harm.
4   Be guided by the potential harm and what is in the patient's best interests against loss of confidentiality, patient respect, dignity and mis-interpretation when using a non-professional interpreter.
5   Remember that the presence of a non-professional interpreter may mean the patient has not disclosed relevant information.

To ensure confidentiality when using video and telephone interpretation services:

1   Video and telephone devices must use hospital-grade encryption processes and calls may not be recorded.
2   All interpreter video stations must be carefully located and not in areas with public access.
3   Similar precautions are required for location of telephone interpreters.

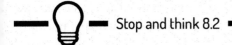 Stop and think 8.2

When you start each placement, ask your practice supervisor if there are Trust or employer guidelines or policies on use of non-professional interpreters. Perhaps there is a local charity that provides interpreters in your area? What problems might you find in maintaining confidentiality using interpreter services and how would you manage this risk?

Dealing with reluctance and resistance

Now we move on to further barriers to delivering care that can come from reluctance, resistance and strong emotions on the part of our patients. Many people may be unwilling to give consent to care and treatment because of fear, moral or personal objection, inability to accept the need (denial of a problem) or inability to understand what is being done to them (Wood et al., 2014). To overcome all of these barriers the practitioner needs good communication skills.

Reluctance

Reluctance often comes about because the person lacks information about the situation and may be expecting worse outcomes than are realistic. A person may withdraw co-operation because they are in pain, disoriented or even embarrassed. Let's look at one example case study.

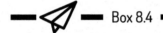 **Box 8.4**

A reluctant patient

A 4-year-old girl has fallen at home and probably broken her wrist. She is in pain and her mother is displaying a lot of anxiety by giving the child lots of attention and fuss. The nurse wants to examine the arm but the child is keeping it firmly tucked under her coat against her chest.

This child is not co-operating because she is fearful of what may happen. Her mother is giving her mixed messages about the seriousness of the situation (by being over-anxious) and this is reinforced by the pain the girl experiences every time she moves her arm. Duxbury (2000) suggests that the communication strategies most useful in cases of fear and anxiety should give support and accurate, clear information and be empathetic and cathartic. Following these guidelines we can suggest in our example that the nurse needs to:

- reduce the child's fear of pain and the mother's anxiety
- reduce the child's expectations of harm
- give realistic information about the situation.

The nurse can do this through communicating:

- the reality of the situation – that the pain is real but won't do major harm
- realistic expectations – that moving the arm will cause pain but this needs to be done to solve the problem
- that both the child and mother can trust the nurse.

Firstly, the nurse should be calm and matter of fact, while being empathetic of the pain experienced. Then, give a simple explanation of the injury, why it hurts and what can be done about it. This is followed by simple but direct and assertive instructions to the child (and the mother) about how and in what way it needs to be examined. The calmness and unflappable, authoritative demeanour of the nurse role-models the level of concern needed (not that much, but something needs to be done to the arm), delivered in a sympathetic but not overly concerned manner. It is important that the right phrases are used to communicate in a reassuring manner, as you can see below.

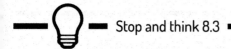 **Stop and think 8.3**

Look at the list below and see which phrases the competent nurse is likely to use in this situation:

1   'Now then, there's no need for all this fuss. It doesn't hurt that much. Let me see it and we can have it fixed in no time.'
2   'I know it hurts; there is probably a small break in there. You need to show me so I can check. I won't touch it but I know it might hurt a bit. The sooner I see it, the sooner we can get it mended.'
3   'Does it hurt a lot? I know, it's not nice is it? It's OK, though; it will mend. You need to show it to me so I can check it and we can stop it hurting.'
4   'Ooh, I bet that hurts! Never mind, it will be better soon. I need to see your arm to get it mended.'

Answer: hopefully, you preferred statements 2 and 3 rather than 1 and 4. Statement 3 is best as it contains reassurance as well as information.

Resistance

Resistance to care could be described as the intentional and deliberate choice of a patient or client to refuse care or engage in the care process. It can be passive or aggressive, manipulative or demanding (Miller, 1990), and can be for a range of reasons that stem from a different set of values around lifestyle choice or treatment approaches (Duxbury, 2000) or, very commonly, fear of losing independence (Konno et al., 2012).

Regardless of the direct reasons, a key problem is a lack of trust in the care practitioner and the treatment or care offered.

Responses to resistance are many and varied, depending on the reasons for resistance, but good communication skills are needed to get to the bottom of the resistance and to facilitate the co-operation of the person. Duxbury (2000) suggests that communication strategies for a resistive patient need to include providing an appropriate environment and relationship (being catalytic), understanding the reasons for the resistance, ensuring privacy, being supportive, rewarding co-operative behaviour and setting firm boundaries.

Look at Practice example box 8.4. This was a real event in which the practitioner needed to address the environmental and nurse–patient relationship barriers and overcome disclosure barriers to assess the care problem.

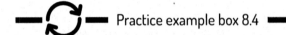 Practice example box 8.4

Overcoming resistance

A specialist drug and alcohol nurse was asked to see an older woman who arrived in the emergency department following a fall. The woman had old and fresh bruises to the outside of her arms suggestive of frequent falls and unsteadiness. Alcohol misuse was suspected but no one tested blood alcohol levels. On initial meeting, the nurse felt that this woman was reluctant to discuss the reasons for her accident as she repeatedly gave obscure and evasive answers. The environment was not at all private, and the woman was dressed in only a backless nightgown and had been moved from a bed to a waiting area.

The nurse found the woman a blanket to cover herself with and moved the interview to the plaster room which was the only unoccupied room that offered privacy. This action helped establish a trusting and co-operative relationship between the nurse and the patient and this environment provided uninterrupted privacy for the nurse to encourage the woman to make disclosures. It became apparent after careful and lengthy interviewing that her husband drank excessively while her own intake was moderate. The patient disclosed that she obtained co-proxamol (an opiate-based analgesic) from her GP for back pain that she didn't have. She was administering the analgesic to her husband without his knowledge, who was otherwise aggressive and probably violent towards her. Her report of his behaviour suggested that he had become dependent on the opiate. She was also being visited by some youths in the neighbourhood who were buying the co-proxamol from her and would threaten her if she didn't give them any.

This interview revealed three important factors about this woman. She was obtaining co-proxamol in order to supply drugs illegally (albeit under duress), she was experiencing domestic violence from her husband and she was using the co-proxamol inappropriately on her husband. These factors had legal, social and health management implications for the woman's life that needed rapid and careful management. If the nurse had not created an environment conducive to a private interview and taken the time to establish and use a trusting relationship with the patient, none of this detail would have been disclosed.

We can summarise that resistance can be caused, and solved, by the points outlined in Table 8.1.

Table 8.1 Managing resistance

Problem	Solution
Patient has incorrect information	Give patient the correct information
Lack of communication of fears by patient	Encourage disclosure of fears
Lack of trust of nurse by patient	Work on the nurse–patient relationship
Patient is worried about a poor outcome	Empower the patient/client to problem-solve

Knowledge link For more details on communication methods with resistance, see Chapters 12 and 15 regarding motivational interviewing.

Dealing with aggression

Data collected in 2017 indicated that 20% of members of staff in mental health or learning disability care environments had experienced violence against them. For all care contexts, nearly 15% of staff experienced violence from patients or their relatives or other members of the public (NHS England, 2019). This evidence helps to emphasise the importance of developing skills in recognising and managing aggressive situations.

Aggression is inevitable and common in certain healthcare situations because it can be a symptom of illness. Therefore, its detection using good observation skills is part of the care assessment process. There are many organic causes of aggression. Common among these are hormonal disturbance, epilepsy, brain tumours, toxic states that cause hallucinations or psychosis (infections or exposure to chemicals), substance withdrawal, dementia, hyperthyroidism, functional psychosis (caused by mental illness) and hypoxia (lack of oxygen to the brain). However, there are also social and environmental causes that health professionals both contribute to and have the ability to manage.

Social and environmental influences of aggression

Certain care settings present greater trigger factors for aggression among patients and relatives than others because of the environment. Apart from care areas such as mental health, dementia and learning difficulty settings, in which aggression is often part of the patient's condition, emergency department have the highest risk for aggression from service users (RCN, 2018).

These settings present some of the typical factors that trigger aggression. In acute care settings, for example, Ferns (2007) identified several factors that contribute to aggression:

- poor communication
- invasive and distressing procedures
- noise
- lack of sleep
- perceived loss of control and powerlessness
- pain
- anxiety
- disorientation.

In certain care situations, anxious patients who are in pain, and relatives who feel helpless, encounter a care environment that involves waiting, lack of attention and poor information-giving, busyness, noise and an alien and disempowering environment which they don't understand. Add to that staff who may be inappropriately chatting about what they did the night before or otherwise ignoring the waiting patients and this causes the potential for a build-up of frustration and anxiety that could turn into aggressive behaviour.

There are many longer-term management strategies that can reduce these triggers for aggression, but in the immediate or short term we need to use good communication to prevent aggression arising or to de-escalate aggression when it occurs.

Firstly, we need to use good observational skills to recognise when a patient is likely to engage in aggressive behaviour. We need to recognise the **prodromal** (before onset of symptoms) signs of aggression such as mounting anxiety, impatience and irritability. Typically, these may be:

- commencement or worsening of stammering
- pacing and staring
- jaw and fist clenching
- defensive posturing (e.g. covering head, standing square-on or raising arms)
- exaggerated gestures and raised voice
- tearfulness (as a result of frustration)

- self-hitting
- withdrawal (becoming silent, uncommunicative or slow to respond).

(Ferns, 2007)

De-escalation principles

Verbal de-escalation is a technique used to reduce potential aggression and should be preferred to any physical management (Spenser et al., 2018). Evidence suggests that de-escalation responses should include a calm, non-confrontational approach, listening to the patient and giving the person a sense of autonomy and their own personal space (Spenser et al., 2018). Adopt a calming tone of voice that is not threatening and do not shout. The nurse is recommended to have an awareness of themselves: be aware of their own body stance (not confrontational), their eye contact (not staring) and of course their own personal safety (Spenser et al., 2018).

To summarise, there are things a nurse can do to disarm the situation:

- adopt a comfortable and relaxed demeanour (avoid 'mirroring' the person's aggressive body language)
- continuously assess the risks to safety
- be genuine and warm
- take time: do not rush the person
- be respectful of the person's views and feelings
- listen actively
- speak clearly, slowly and in short sentences
- maintain a large personal space (for the nurse and the person concerned!).

In doing the above, the nurse is then in a position to engage the person in conversation about their feelings without them feeling threatened. There are some sensible communication strategies that the nurse can adopt to reduce the person's strong emotions:

- encourage the person to talk and identify the problem
- avoid disagreeing or saying that you know how they feel (you don't)
- describe what has been happening (give the person the information they need)
- identify and suggest possible coping strategies, if possible (e.g. getting some fresh air outside, phoning a friend or getting a cup of tea from the canteen)
- provide ways of resolving the situation, if possible.

In the event of actual aggression or violence, the student nurse is not expected to manage the situation. Specific training in dealing with aggression is only given to qualified staff. In the case of actual aggression, the only course of action for the student is to get out of the situation and call for help. If a student nurse finds themself in a situation that threatens to become violent, the student must remove themself from the situation and ask staff to intervene.

Conclusion

This chapter has attempted to address some of the challenges to communication that are not dealt with specifically in other chapters in this book, but are likely to present themselves in all branches of nursing. The home visit deprives the nurse of the power of the institution and demands skills in assertiveness and management of the environment. The use of interpreters is becoming more common in a world where borders have become flexible to workers, visitors and refugees, and where immigration represents a major social change to the society. The ability to work effectively with interpreters is likely to become increasingly important to nurses in a future where global mobility is increasing. Use of technology in this regard has been found to be of great help.

This chapter has also addressed the basic knowledge and skills for dealing with aggression which, like a language barrier, demands effective communication skills from nursing staff. This can be a specialised area of nursing, particularly in mental health and when working with people with learning difficulties, but applies to all nurses and in many areas and environments of healthcare.

Communication challenges can often be unique. No two situations are exactly the same, but by applying the basic skills we can negotiate our way through most of the common challenges.

FURTHER READING

Holland, K. (2016) *Cultural Awareness in Nursing and Healthcare: An Introductory Text.* London, Routledge.

REFERENCES

Bond, M. and Pearson, K. (1969) Psychological aspects of pain in women with advanced carcinoma of the cervix. *Journal of Psychosomatic Research*, 13, 13–19.

Burnett, A. and Peel, M. (2001) Health needs of asylum seekers and refugees. *British Medical Journal*, 322, 544–577.

DeVito, J. (1988) *Human Communication: The Basic Course* (4th edn). New York, Harper & Row.

Duxbury, J. (2000) *Difficult Patients*. Oxford, Butterworth Heinemann.

Ferns, T. (2007) Factors that influence aggressive behaviour in acute care settings. *Nursing Standard*, 21(33), 41–45.

Hadziabdic, E., Albin, B., Heikkila, K. and Hjelm, K. (2014) Family members' experiences of the use of interpreters in healthcare. *Primary Health Care Research & Development*, 15, 156–169.

Halliday, T. (1992) Touch and pain. In T. Halliday (ed.), *The Senses and Communication* (pp. 147–210). Buckingham, Open University Press.

Holland, K. and Hogg, C. (2010) *Cultural Awareness in Nursing and Healthcare* (2nd edn). London, Hodder Education.

Houghton, M. (2016) *Culture and Society Defined*. www.cliffsnotes.com/study-guides/sociology/culture-and-societies/culture-and-society-defined (accessed 13 February 2019).

Kang, C., Farrington, R. and Tomkow, L. (2019) Access to primary health care for asylum seekers and refugees: a qualitative study of service user experiences in the UK. *British Journal of General Practice*, bjgp19X701309. doi: 10.3399/bjgp19X701309.

Konno, R., Kang, H.S. and Makimoto, K. (2012) The best evidence for minimizing resistance-to-care during assisted personal care for older adults with dementia in nursing homes: a systematic review. *JBI Library of Systematic Reviews*, 10(58), 4622–4632.

Masland, M.C., Lou, C. and Snowden, L. (2010) Use of communication technologies to cost-effectively increase the availability of interpretation services in healthcare settings. *Telemedicine Journal and e-Health*, 16(6), 739–745.

Miller, R. (1990) *Managing Difficult Patients*. London, Faber & Faber.

NHS England (2019) *NHS Staff Survey 2018: National Results Briefing*. London, NHS England.

NMC (2010) *Standards for Pre-registration Nursing Education: Draft for Consultation*. London, Nursing and Midwifery Council.

NMC (2018) *Future Nurse: Standards of Proficiency for Registered Nurses*. www.nmc.org.uk/globalassets/sitedocuments/education-standards/future-nurse-proficiencies.pdf.

Osae-Larbi, J.A. (2016) Bridging the language barrier gap in the health of multicultural societes: report of a proposed mobile phone-based intervention using Ghana as an example. *SpringerPlus*, 5(1), 900.

RCN (2018) *Violence and Aggression in the NHS Estimating the Size and the Impact of the Problem: Interim Report*. London, Royal College of Nursing.

Spencer, S., Johnson, P. and Smith, I.C. (2018) De-escalation techniques for managing non-psychosis induced aggression in adults (Review). *Cochrane Database of Systematic Reviews*, 7, CD012034.

Tribe, R. (2007) Working with interpreters. *The Psychologist*, 20(3), 159–161.

Wood, F., Martin, S.M, Carson-Stevens, A., Elwyn, G., Precious, E. and Kinnersley, P. (2014) Doctors' perspectives of informed consent for non-emergency surgical procedures: a qualitative interview study. *Health Expectations*, 19, 751–761.

Yu-Hsin, K.L., Henceroth, M., Lu, Q. and LeRoy, A. (2016) Cultural differences in pain experience among four ethnic groups: a qualitative pilot study. *Journal of Behavioral Health*, 5(2), 75–81.

NINE
HEALTH PROMOTION AND COMMUNICATION TECHNIQUES

MAXINE HOLT AND LUCY WEBB

.... THIS CHAPTER WILL HELP YOU TO:

- Promote health and wellbeing, self-care and independence
- Provide appropriate advice and guidance to individuals, communities and populations
- Work within a public health framework to assess needs and plan care

Introduction

In 1891, Florence Nightingale stated,

> I look forward to the day when there will be no nurses of the sick, only nurses of
> the well.

(Nightingale, 1891)

Of course, we can interpret Florence Nightingale's meaning in the context of that particular era, although if we were to consider it from a health promotion and prevention perspective in the twenty-first century, she might be encouraged to see that the role of the nurse is increasingly one of health promotion and illness prevention. This is recognised as such by the NMC (2018a). Also, healthcare in England, as delivered by *The NHS Long Term Plan* (NHS England, 2019), focuses more attention on preventing illness and encouraging a greater degree of self-help by the population as a whole. This puts nurses at the heart of face-to-face health promotion to the patients, families and members of the public we encounter in our professional lives.

This chapter will explore the different levels and methods we use to communicate health messages to the different groups in our nursing role. It will examine the different settings we work in as nurses and how they may be used to communicate health promotion across a diverse range of patients.

The NMC (2018a) has health promotion as a key standard of proficiency and requires nurses to:

> understand and apply the aims and principles of health promotion, protection and improvement and the prevention of ill health when engaging with people.
>
> (NMC, 2018a:11)

This requirement is about enabling positive health and wellbeing by reducing individual risk factors, for example physical inactivity, poor diet and nutrition, and strengthening protective factors, such as smoking cessation. But it also incorporates wider socioeconomic and environmental factors, for example poverty.

Nurse health promoters need to be competent in a number of skills, and effective communication is one which we all need to develop. As a nurse you will meet a lot of patients who have diverse health promotion needs which are influenced by many factors. These may include culture, sex, age, educational attainment or perhaps a chronic physical or mental illness. Effective communication in promoting health and wellbeing ensures that health promotion interventions are tailored to meet the different needs of our patients.

Individual and population levels of communication in promoting health

Firstly, we need to think about the different levels we use to communicate health promotion as nurses. Think back to the point above regarding the range of health promotion campaigns and how they are communicated. We can see that such campaigns can occur on a large scale, targeting the population in general or, alternatively, they may be aimed at specific organisations, groups or individuals. Consider the NHS England (2018) flu vaccine campaign poster in Figure 9.1. Do you consider this to be a means of communicating a health promotion message to individuals or groups?

It is a very familiar campaign that we see occurring each year around October and through the winter months to protect people against current strains of flu. It is communicated to the general public by NHS England and aims to reach particular at-risk groups in society. Nurses are very much involved in communicating the campaign to patients on an individual basis and do this in a variety of ways. For example, a

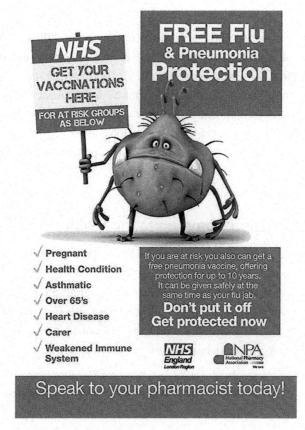

Figure 9.1 Flu and pneumonia vaccine campaign poster

Source: Crown copyright

practice nurse may discuss the need for a patient to consider the vaccine during a routine clinic visit to the asthma clinic:

'Well, John, your asthma symptoms are really well under control at the moment but winter is a tricky time for anyone who has asthma so you might want to consider having a flu jab to protect you. Have a look at this leaflet, which explains a little more about it and if you have any questions ask me. If you decide that you want to have the vaccine, we can do it today so that you don't need to make another appointment'.

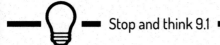 Stop and think 9.1

Can you think of other ways in which nurses can communicate the message to patients? Some suggestions are detailed in this chapter.

Nurses working in other areas such as in outpatient departments or on medical wards can provide at-risk patients with the necessary information and direct the patient to the appropriate means of receiving the vaccine. Children's nurses may provide parents with advice on vaccinations for measles or meningitis. The point is that nurses are in a position to communicate health promotion from community level through to individual level. This will be dependent upon our nursing role or area of work but it is important to consider that we are able to communicate health promotion in a variety of ways. This may be by working with patients or by designing, planning and influencing health promotion campaigns or policies.

Nurses as role models in communicating health

Another way that practitioners can promote health to patients is as role models for the patients and communities we serve (Darch et al., 2017). However, the idea of nurses acting as role models causes strong disagreement among some nurses (Wills et al., 2019). Our own research (Box 9.1) has revealed that nurses are reluctant to discuss topics with patients that might be challenging for both the patient and the nurse; for example, smoking, particularly if the nurse is a smoker.

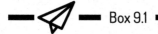 Box 9.1

Practitioner comments

I wouldn't suggest to patients that they need to give up smoking because I'm a smoker and I'd feel that I was being a hypocrite. (Nurse's quote)

How can I really discuss or ask a patient about their alcohol intake when we go out at weekends and probably drink more than the recommended amount? (Nurse's quote)

(Holt, 2008)

Wills et al.'s (2019) research found that overweight nurses were reluctant to conform to healthy behaviours in order to be healthy role models. It can therefore be too high an expectation on nurses. However, being seen to be 'human' can also be a positive characteristic (Kelly et al., 2017) and may help us to empathise better with our patients.

Where and when is health promotion communicated?

The UK health policy Making Every Contact Count is an evidence-based strategy that aims to tackle lifestyle diseases by targeting behaviour change. It charges all public sector organisations to make a positive impact on physical and mental health and well-being (Health Education England, 2019). This approach recognises that our everyday contacts with the public offer an opportunity to deliver information and motivation to our patients to encourage a healthier lifestyle. This might be relating to increasing the amount of exercise taken, stopping smoking, eating healthily or reducing alcohol consumption. For health practitioners, health promotion does not need to be restricted to healthcare settings.

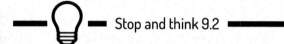

Stop and think 9.2

Before you look at the suggested list below, make your own list of as many settings as you can where health promotion can be communicated.

Health promotion can be communicated both inside and outside the NHS and below are some settings that you might have included in your list:

Educational: schools, colleges, universities, pre-school nurseries, after-school clubs

Healthcare and social care: hospitals, dentists, primary care surgeries, police stations, NHS walk-in centres, elderly care homes, pharmacists, polyclinics, prisons

Social/environmental: pubs, nightclubs, supermarkets, workplaces, neighbourhoods, churches, gyms, over-60s clubs, red-light districts, homeless shelters

The above are just a few examples and the list of settings has become a global initiative. One of the advantages of using different settings is that it enables problems to be tackled with a holistic approach. Another advantage is that it enables us to communicate with those who are often difficult to reach, such as the young, the disadvantaged or those who are marginalised in some way.

A problem with targeted health promotion is that people can feel stigmatised (Corcoran and Bone, 2007). For example, targeting obesity may make obese people feel ashamed. If you consider the above list there are many venues which offer the nurse an opportunity to be involved in communicating about health.

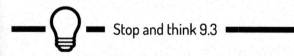

Stop and think 9.3

Think about your own area of nursing work or a recent practice placement you have experienced and identify the opportunities you have/had for communicating health promotion.

You might have initially considered your first contact with a patient or family and how you both began the process of assessment of their needs and subsequent planning of care to meet those needs. It may be that when you prepared a patient due for discharge, they needed advice on how to take their medication or how to access other services for the continuation of their care. Another example is during a procedure, such as a dressing or assisting with personal hygiene or when teaching someone a skill; for example, administration of insulin to someone newly diagnosed with diabetes. A school nurse will be involved in screening programmes and providing health education sessions to children, teachers and parents. Occupational health nurses are involved in providing advice and communicating with the workforce and the managers on health issues.

As you can see, the opportunities across different settings are vast and it is important to remember that communication in health promotion may not always be directly to patients. Health promotion involves communicating and working with other partners and stakeholders to develop health promotion initiatives, developing or directing policy and providing written papers and other documents. As nurses we are very much involved in such areas and need to acquire good communication skills for a diverse range of situations.

How is health promotion communicated?

So far, we have explored how nurses can deliver health promotion across a range of opportunities, at different levels and in various settings. Let's now consider the different methods used and how we can develop these methods. The use of mass media is perhaps the most popular and a frequently used method to provide information about health issues and promote behaviour change. Mass media is a powerful means of communication and just to give you an example of how powerful it can be, listen to the following broadcast on YouTube: www.youtube.com/watch?v=YTvU9j3og5k.

Obviously, this was not a health promotion campaign although it did have a significant effect on the wellbeing of some 1 million people for a short time on 10 October 1938. It is in fact a clip of the radio broadcast of the H.G. Wells sci-fi story *War of The Worlds*. Such was the power of the story and the way in which it was communicated that it is estimated that 1 million people fled their homes in terror as they believed that the world was being invaded by aliens.

Many Flee Homes to Escape 'Gas Raid from Mars'—Phone Calls Swamp Police at Broadcast of Wells Fantasy.

(This article appeared in the *New York Times* on 31 October 1938)

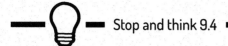
Stop and think 9.4

Can you think of some examples from health promotion which may be said to have had similar effects? See suggestions in the text below.

Modern-day examples of widespread effects from health promotion can be identified as those relating to early campaigns on HIV and AIDS, or the current concerns with obesity and type 2 diabetes. Many patients and their families will access their health information via mass media and nurses need to be able to recognise the influence that this may have on their beliefs about, and ability to act upon, such information. There is a range of mass media forms that enable health promoters such as nurses to reach out to individuals and even whole populations. Table 9.1 shows four categories of mass media adapted from Corcoran and Bone (2007) and how they may be applied to health promotion.

Table 9.1 Categories of mass media and their application to health promotion

Type of media	Example	Ways to use media	Ways nurses may use the media to communicate health promotion
Audiovisual, broadcast	Television, radio	News, documentaries, soap operas, advertisements, public announcements	
Audiovisual, non-broadcast	DVD, CD, downloadable podcasts	Self-help packages, teaching packages	
Printed material	Newspapers, magazines, journals, leaflets, booklets, billboards, posters, games	Advertisements, news items, stories, magazine features	
Electronic material	Online, phone, social media	YouTube, text messaging, apps, podcasts, websites, online learning	

Source: adapted from Corcoran and Bone (2007)

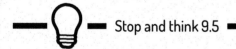
Stop and think 9.5

The fourth column of Table 9.1 has been left blank for you to consider how you might use the suggested media in your nursing role. Complete the column, giving examples of how you may apply this form of communication in your health promotion work. Then see Table 9.2 for suggestions.

One of the important features of the mass media is that it has a role in educating people through information-giving or entertainment, providing or clarifying meanings for people about health topics and influencing behaviour and lifestyle. The use of the mass media to communicate health is one which underpins the goals of health promotion. These are to provide evidence-based, objective information to the patients and families we work with and to contribute to policy development. Let us now consider some of the examples you may have given in the previous exercise.

Table 9.2 Categories of mass media and ways that nurses can use them in health promotion

Type of media	Example	Ways nurses may use the media to communicate health promotion
Audiovisual, broadcast	Television, radio	Public announcements, i.e. the flu vaccine campaign on local radio. Local initiatives identified as part of local delivery plans, i.e. screening services or well persons clinics. School plays which represent a particular theme, e.g. drug misuse.
Audiovisual, non-broadcast	DVD, CD, downloadable podcasts	Self-help packages for newly diagnosed diabetics, asthmatics. Educational CDs on specific conditions such as autism. Relaxation therapies and techniques for stress management.
Printed material	Newspapers, magazines, journals, leaflets, booklets, billboards, posters, games	Leaflets on healthy eating or other lifestyle and health behaviours. Patient newsletters, i.e. stroke club or local breathe-easy group. Posters on current health topics or services available.
Electronic material	Online, phone, social media	NHS Live Well website, self-help apps, patient-run websites, YouTube education videos, chat rooms, Facebook, etc.

Source: adapted from Corcoran and Bone (2007)

The opportunities for nurses to use mass media to communicate health are very broad indeed and Table 9.2 provides just a few examples. Whether we choose online resources or physical resources such as booklets may depend on the setting. For example, a leaflet is easy to give to someone in a brief intervention, while an online resource in the public domain can be accessible to anyone who looks for it.

Social media has been found to be empowering for patients and often improves the relationship with healthcare professionals (Smailhodzic et al., 2016), but we need to recognise that there are some problems with using any mass media to communicate health promotion. It can be very expensive, a fact nurses would need to consider if planning any campaigns, and inaccurate information from unregulated sources can give people a false impression that there are simple cures or untested treatments available. We need to be able to support patients whose health and wellbeing is influenced by what they read or hear in the media by giving accurate, evidence-based and objective information. In addition, we must appreciate that such materials should, wherever possible, be used to reinforce verbal information, and be appropriate to the person. See Practice example box 9.1.

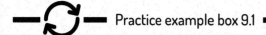 Practice example box 9.1

Health promotion and learning disability

Well done, Joan, you have named a lot of food today that will help you lose weight. You can try using this leaflet that has good pictures of foods you can try, too.

Patient information leaflets have been shown to support patients' knowledge and improve satisfaction with treatment and treatment adherence (Sustersic et al., 2017). There are some other important factors, though, that we need to consider when using information materials to communicate health promotion.

Treadgold and Grant's review of the evidence (2014:6–7) indicates three key areas for effective health information for patients (see Box 9.2).

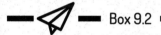 Box 9.2

Three factors for effective health information

Relevance:

- meets patient's needs
- tailored and personalised information.

Accuracy:

- accurate, evidence-based, transparent
- unbiased communication of risks, benefits and uncertainties
- involves healthcare experts in its development.

Readability:

- keeps language and numbers simple, communicated clearly
- breaks down complex information
- lays out information to aid navigation
- uses visually attractive materials.

Let's look at these themes in more detail.

Relevance and readability

We need to ensure that the materials are suitable for our patients and a recommended way to do this is simply involve patients in the conception and design of health information. Patient and public involvement in healthcare has been developing in many countries and in the UK is acknowledged to be vital to ensuring that services develop to meet patient needs (National Institute for Health Research, 2015). Consultation with a patient group will ensure that material is relevant to their needs as well as addressing readability. The Ewles and Simnett approach to health promotion (Scriven, 2017) suggests further advice for nurses to consider when designing health promotion resources which could be used in conjunction with patient consultation:

- Is the resource appropriate for achieving the intended aims?
- Would another type of medium be better?
- Is the information clear and to the point?
- Are the key themes emphasised?
- Does the resource communicate the message in a language which is easily understood by the patient or their family?
- Does the resource look appealing?

Accuracy

Some information can be confusing for patients simply because it can change so often.

It is important that the information we communicate to patients and their families is current and underpinned by sound evidence. As nurses we need to be able to direct patients to sources of good quality health information, including health-related websites.

Some website examples you might want to use are:

http://easyhealth.org.uk/

www.mind.org.uk/information-support/

www.nhs.uk/common-health-questions/childrens-health/

www.nhs.uk/live-well/

www.patient.co.uk/

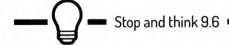 Stop and think 9.6

In advance of your next placement, look at the websites listed above to see what information is available on the health conditions or issues you are likely to encounter, as well as information for any health promotion opportunities which may arise. When you arrive on placement, ask your practice facilitator and colleagues to direct you to other resources they have.

Let's look critically at another example and see if it is meeting Treadgold and Grant's three key criteria.

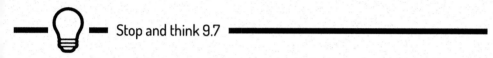

Stop and think 9.7

Look again at the NHS England flu and pneumonia vaccine campaign poster in Figure 9.1. How do you think it addresses the three themes of relevance, accuracy and readability?

We can see that the use of the poster for this topic area is *relevant* for the targeted at-risk population. It is *accurate*, emphasising key points, and is likely to be evidence-based. The information is brief and to the point and the poster is certainly eye-catching, using the theme of a nasty bug to emphasise the seriousness of the message in a simple, *readable* way.

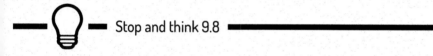

Stop and think 9.8

Consider another aspect of health promotion which may need communicating to the general public to address or raise local health agendas. How might you do this? See the text below to see if you are on the right lines.

You may have thought of outbreaks of measles or chicken pox, perhaps a bad batch of an illegal substance that drug users might use or a high rate of obesity in the locality. One of the ways in which nurses can use the local press is through the use of stories on health topics which depict a positive message, such as success stories addressing a local issue (remembering confidentiality and data protection issues). Other ways are through letters or articles in the local primary care practice or the Primary Care Trust newsletter. Communicating health promotion is also about working across disciplines and other agencies and relies on good communication skills in working with other partners.

Factors that influence health communication

We have so far considered the different methods that nurses can use to communicate health promotion. We now need to consider some of the factors which may influence health and help people to act upon health promotion. Health is influenced by a multitude of complex factors which include local and national policy, living environments, socio-economic status, work and genetics. It is important then that we are aware of such factors and are able to take these into consideration when communicating health promotion, both with patients and other stakeholders. It is also worth noting that in the broader sense of health promotion work we are more likely to gain resources and financial support if our interventions are in line with current policy, at a national and local level. Figure 9.2 represents a simple model of the influences on the individual and their health. The individual's health factors could be age, sex and genes that shape their health potential. These are often referred to as non-modifiable factors: factors that the individual cannot change. Alongside these, however, are modifiable behaviours such as smoking, the level of exercise taken and diet. Surrounding the individual are factors such as the family and immediate culture the person belongs to that can promote or damage health. Among these we could include ethnicity and class. Alongside there are social and community influences such as education level, urban or rural living and economic power (for instance income, ability to travel and the use of private healthcare) which may have a positive or negative effect. Beyond these is the sociopolitical environment which we can regard as national-level influencers, for instance regulation of cigarette advertising, food labelling or drink-driving laws.

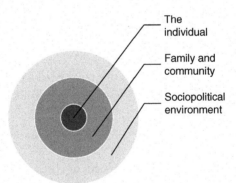

Figure 9.2 Influences on health and wellbeing

Barton and Grant (2006) suggest that the links between the community and sustainability of healthy communities are fundamental in promoting health and wellbeing. In order to consider how we may communicate health promotion let us begin by considering social factors which may influence our patients.

━━○━ Stop and think 9.9 ━━━━━━━━━━

What social factors would you need to consider when using the flu vaccine poster to communicate the need for vaccination to the patients below?

- A 70-year-old with coronary heart disease
- An 8-year-old child with asthma

See the following text for answers.

There are several things we would need to consider, for example the age range of our patients will influence how they are able to apply, interpret and react to language. If we look at the above example, we can see that how we describe the problem of not having the vaccine will vary between age groups. Older adults are likely to be able to access the written information on the poster, while children will love the graphics which tell the story of nasty bugs that cause disease.

One word of caution is not to assume that all patients in each age range will respond in the same way. We need to remember that this may be affected by other factors such as physical, cognitive or mental disability or impairment. Age and gender also influence how we interpret health promotion messages and how we want to be communicated with. The patients we work with will come from different social classes, and have a variety of educational attainment levels. These are factors which will influence the ability of patients to respond to and understand health messages. Ethnicity and culture are also important factors in communication in health promotion. Another point to note is not to assume that all patients who do not have English as their first language automatically read their own language. Many may speak their first language at home but not read it. Other factors such as the attitudes and beliefs of our patients are also influencing factors in communication, and there are a number of theoretical models which seek to predict responses to these in an effort to change behaviour.

....

Knowledge link Theoretical models are discussed in more detail in Chapter 15 of this book.

....

Using nursing assessment to communicate health promotion

We have considered the use of different resources that nurses can use to communicate health promotion, and now need to consider how we can use our own nursing assessment tools for the same means. A contemporary understanding of Florence Nightingale's theory of health and illness suggests that one of our most important jobs is to ensure that the patient is placed in the correct circumstances to ensure their optimal health and wellbeing. In order to do this, we are required to develop a sound knowledge base, and skills in observation and communication to assess, inform and educate patients and their families (NMC, 2018b).

Many nurses have the skills which enable them to incorporate health promotion principles into their existing work, and this is in line with current government and nursing policy (NMC, 2018a; NHS England, 2019). The theoretical principles that underpin the nursing assessment are those of a gateway for the building of the nurse–patient relationship to enable assessment of the patient's needs and goal-setting. Within this ideology the opportunity to assess health and wellbeing and initiate health promotion interventions is perhaps an inevitable part of the process.

The theory that underpins the patient assessment is that it presents an opportunity for the nurse to develop a relationship with the patient in order to assess their needs, set goals and plan interventions to meet those goals. It is a significant opportunity for the nurse to engage in communicating with the patient about their health and wellbeing and offer advice and support where and if necessary. Let us now consider then how we may use the nursing assessment to communicate health promotion.

There are many theoretical nursing models which we can use to guide our nursing practice and which we use will depend upon the particular area of nursing we work in. The Roper, Logan and Tierney model of nursing (1983) is based on Activities of Daily Living that every person needs to be able to perform. These are as follows:

- maintaining a safe environment
- communicating
- breathing
- eating and drinking
- eliminating
- personal cleansing and dressing

- controlling body temperature
- mobilising
- working and playing
- expressing sexuality
- sleeping
- dying.

Many of the nursing assessment documents that you will see and use in practice are designed to reflect these Activities of Daily Living. The model enables the nurse to not only assess the actual problems the patient may have but also place emphasis on prevention and health promotion. As a nurse you will, at some stage, spend time with a patient discussing their problems, from which you will jointly develop a plan of care. It is during this process that you may be able to begin a dialogue with the patient about a health issue. See Practice example box 9.2.

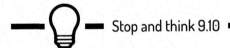 **Stop and think 9.10**

Look at Practice example box 9.2. Can you identify any opportunities for using the nursing assessment to communicate health promotion for Mr D?

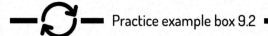 Practice example box 9.2

Assessment opportunities for health promotion

Mr D is 60 and of Pakistani origin. He arrives on the ward from the emergency department after having a dizzy spell. This occurred following a fall at home while getting up to go to the toilet during the night. This is something which he says he often has to do. He has just retired from being a taxi driver due to ill health. He has type 2 diabetes and is hypertensive and obese. He takes diuretics and anti-hypertensive therapy, although occasionally he forgets to take his medication, and has a regular blood pressure of 150/100 mmHg. He and his wife are due to go on a Haj pilgrimage to Mecca within the next week.

The following is not a complete assessment of Mr D's needs but suggests examples of how nurses can use the nursing assessment to communicate health promotion. It must be stressed that this is an integrative process and that health needs also reflect those which aim to promote and protect health and wellbeing in addition to those which may present as immediate or existing problems. See Table 9.3.

Table 9.3 Mr D's likely needs

Activities of Daily Living	Health promotion opportunity
Maintaining a safe environment and personal cleansing and dressing	Medication advice: Mr D fell while getting up to use the toilet during the night. He takes diuretics and quite often patients do not follow the directions on the medication. He may therefore be taking his diuretic in the evening rather than the morning, resulting in him having to get up often during the night.
	Foot care advice: Both he and his wife are going to Mecca in the near future. This can involve walking in bare feet. The feet of a diabetic patient are very prone to injury which can have devastating effects.
Communicating, eating and drinking and mobilising	Consider the need for an interpreter if necessary: patients who do not have English as their first language may often not comply with instructions and may not understand colloquial terms that we may use.
	Discuss the need to maintain healthy body weight and its relationship to high blood pressure: promote healthy eating and perhaps involve Mrs D in discussion. Refer to dietitian.
	Teach how to take and record and interpret own blood pressure: involving Mr D in management of his own blood pressure, record-keeping and when to consult for further advice.
	Provide leaflet and audio CD in Urdu on foot care and diet for diabetics: Mr D may or may not read Urdu so check first. He may find an audio version useful. Give him these while he is on the ward so that he can read or listen to them and then ask further questions if necessary.

We can use the assessment process as a means of getting to know and understand the patients we work with. It facilitates a discussion with the patients on the factors that influence their health and wellbeing and opens up opportunities to use this information to communicate health promotion.

Conclusion

This chapter has enabled you to consider the different levels at which health promotion is communicated and the different settings in which you may communicate health promotion. It has helped you to recognise that communicating health promotion occurs both in primary and secondary care and at the community and individual levels. The key to successful communication in health promotion is to take the core principles of communication and apply them to health promotion while appreciating the diversity of the patients and people we work with in promoting health.

FURTHER READING

NHS England. *NHS Long Term Plan*. www.longertermplan.nhs.uk/
Patient Platform. *Patient Information*. www.patient.co.uk/
Royal College of Nursing. *Promoting Health*. http://rcni/com/hosted-content/rcn/first-steps/
  promoting-health

REFERENCES

Barton, H. and Grant, M. (2006) A health map for the local human habitat. *Journal of the Royal Society for the Promotion of Health*, 126, 252–253.

Corcoran, N. and Bone, A. (2007) Using settings to communicate health promotion. In N. Corcoran (ed.), *Communicating Health: Strategies for Health Promotion* (pp. 117–138). London, SAGE Publications.

Darch, J., Baillie, L. and Gillison, F. (2017) Nurses as role models in health promotion: a concept analysis. *British Journal of Nursing*, 26(17), 982–988.

Health Education England (2019) *Making Every Contact Count*. www. makingeverycontactcount.co.uk/ (accessed 10 January 2018).

Holt, M. (2008) The educational preparation of student nurses as communicators of health and wellbeing. *The Journal of The Royal Society for the Promotion of Health*, 128(4), 159–160.

Kelly, M., Wills, J.D., Jester, R. and Speller, V. (2017) Should nurses be role models for healthy lifestyles? Results from a modified Delphi study. *Journal of Advanced Nursing*, 73(3), 665–678.

National Institute for Health Research (2015) *Going the extra mile: improving the nation's health and wellbeing through public involvement in research*. www.nihr.ac.uk/patients-and-public/documents/Going-the-Extra-Mile.pdf (accessed 12 January 2019).

NHS England (2018) *NHS-led Flu Campaign*. www.england.nhs.uk/nhsidentity/examples/nhs-led-flu-campaign-with-supporting-partners-poster/ (accessed 9 January 2019).

NHS England (2019) *The NHS Long Term Plan*. London, NHS England.

Nightingale, F. (1891) *Notes on Nursing: What It Is and What It Is Not*. London, Harrison.

NMC (2018a) *Future Nurse: Standards of Proficiency for Registered Nurses*. www.nmc.org.uk/globalassets/sitedocuments/education-standards/future-nurse-proficiencies.pdf.

NMC (2018b) *The Code: Professional Standards of Practice and Behaviour for Nurses, Midwives and Nursing Associates*. www.nmc.org.uk/standards/code/.

Roper, N., Logan, W. and Tierney, A. (1983) *Using a Model for Nursing*. Edinburgh, Churchill Livingstone.

Scriven, A. (2017) *Ewles & Simnett's Promoting Health: A Practical Guide* (7th edn). London, Elsevier.

Smailhodzic, E., Hooijsma, W., Boonstra, A. and Langley, D. (2016) Social media use in healthcare: a systematic review of effects on patients and on their relationship with healthcare professionals. *BMC Health Services Research*, 16, 442.

Sustersic, M., Gauchet, A., Foote, A. and Bosson, J.-L. (2017) How best to use and evaluate Patient Information Leaflets given during a consultation: a systematic review of literature reviews. *Health Expectations*, 20, 531–542.

Treadgold, P. and Grant, C. (2014) *Evidence Review: What Does Good Health Information Look Like?* Patient Information Forum, London. www.pifonline.org.uk/wp-content/uploads/2015/03/What-does-good-health-information-look-like-October-2014.pdf (accessed 12 January 2019).

Wills, J., Kelly, M. and Frings, D. (2019) Nurses as role models in health promotion: piloting the acceptability of a social marketing campaign. *Journal of Advanced Nursing*, 75, 423–431.

TEN
PROFESSIONAL COMMUNICATION SKILLS FOR STUDENT SURVIVAL: SELF-MANAGEMENT, WRITING AND PRESENTING

LUCY WEBB

.... THIS CHAPTER WILL HELP YOU TO:

- Communicate effectively, orally and in writing, so that the meaning is always clear
- Record information accurately and clearly
- Communicate people's stated needs and wishes to other professionals
- Provide accurate and comprehensive written and verbal reports based on the best available evidence

Introduction

This chapter aims to help you manage the journey from novice student to professional nurse, in the way you communicate with colleagues in the academic and practice environments. As a student nurse you will have to acquire skills to support your studies, and develop personal and professional communication skills to practise effectively. Therefore, this chapter will look at meeting challenges in practice, including personal resilience and stress, learning and writing skills for clinical and academic writing, and making presentations.

The challenges facing the student nurse

A lot of communication advice for the student nurse aims to develop professional skills with patients and relatives, for example by developing the nurse–patient relationship and applying active listening skills. While this is incredibly important, there are broader communication skills that help the student nurse develop as a person in a professional setting and reduce the stress of the learning experience.

Healthcare is a high-pressure profession to enter because it involves dealing with people who are stressed, distressed and demanding. For nursing students, key sources of stress come from the academic work and workload, from clinical experiences and personal problems during training (Pulido-Martos et al., 2012). Being effective in such an environment requires personal skills as well as professional ones to meet the demands of the job. All health students go through a process of 'professional socialisation' into the role of the professional (Mackintosh, 2006). This is stressful in itself as old aspects of oneself are discarded and new characteristics are adopted. Any nurse can tell you that training to be a nurse changes people. A person finishing a nurse education programme will be very different to the one who started. Along the way, many new personal skills have to be acquired and practised. Let's consider some that you will encounter.

The nurse role and developing resilience

On your first placement as a student you may have already experienced being called 'nurse'. When you adopt the nurse role, and put on the uniform, you the person have become you the nurse. People have greater expectations of nurses; they expect a particular type of behaviour that would be extraordinary in any other context. To adapt to that level of expectation, the student has to 'become' that person while in the nurse role. This can be very uncomfortable if that role is not like our real selves at all. For example, you may be expected to be dynamic and active and lead a social sing-song for older residential patients, even though you are really a quiet, thoughtful person, or hold a stranger's hand while they cry, despite such intimacy being quite alien to you. At these times, we discover the difference between the nurse 'role' and our personal identity – when we are out of our comfort zone.

Student nurses need to be supported in developing resilience to personal stresses that come with the job. Murray (2014) suggests that resilience to stress is a personal trait that nurse students can develop during training. Resilience is linked positively with emotional intelligence, so that developing emotional intelligence increases one's resilience to stress (Nightingale et al., 2018). Emotional intelligence is still an evolving concept but Goleman (2004) suggests that it can be characterised as:

- self-awareness
- self-regulation

- motivation
- empathy
- social skill.

Check out Goleman's 2004 article on emotional intelligence for details on all these components from the References list at the end of this chapter. The important components here, however, are self-awareness and social skill.

You will have seen in earlier chapters how reflection and self-exploration help develop self-awareness, and knowledge of the dynamics of communication enables nurses to better understand other people's emotional states and how to best respond to them. So reflective practice, self-development and improving communication skills lead to better emotional intelligence and resilience.

The NMC standards for nurse education (NMC, 2018a) support the empowerment of student nurses in order to develop resilience during training and ensure students access the best available experiences for learning. Reflection is championed by the NMC as a key self-development tool, as is the right to be given positive and accurate feedback, pastoral support and adjustments to learning if required. This makes a positive change to the nursing training regulations that recognises the value of students as advocates for patients and champions of the profession they are entering. It also underpins the leadership role of the next generation of nurses by promoting self-development, resilience-building and professionalism. As a student nurse, you should be experiencing encouragement to think for yourself and become an informed and active learner.

Working with others

Most healthcare professionals work as a team. That means working with people we sometimes don't like, don't gel with or even can't stand. Nevertheless, the professional needs to separate their personal values from their professional values and judge the situation in terms of effectiveness for the patient, rather than what should or shouldn't happen according to a personal viewpoint.

Conflict with other people in our teams is inevitable. It might be a clash of personalities or a professional difference in opinion or approach. Either way, it is very difficult to 'get on with the job' unless we develop some personal strategies in the way we communicate with our colleagues that separate the 'professional' persona from our own identity.

Becoming a confident practitioner

Many students say that their biggest challenge is becoming confident in practice. Studies have shown, however, that this is natural and does not mean they are not competent or that their confidence won't develop (Lauder et al., 2008; Thomson et al., 2017). There are many situations that can deflate a student's confidence in the practice setting, just as there are situations that can boost confidence. However, a student will put themselves in the way of new challenges all the time, so it is inevitable that many situations and events will be new, unexpected and difficult, and often lead to unsatisfactory outcomes. That is the learning process.

This process is about communication because it is related to personal development and maturity. How we communicate with others is influenced by our self-confidence and assuredness in what we are doing. Therefore, the student's confidence needs to grow in order to communicate professionally and effectively at each stage of the learning process. An essential skill to learn for any health professional is how to manage stress effectively. Here we will focus on the techniques and skills that involve communication specifically.

Managing stress: using communication skills

The obvious technique in managing your own stress is to communicate with other people. A problem shared, as the proverb goes, is a problem halved. Well, up to a point. It depends who you share it with and how. But let's look at this.

There are some simple 'rules' that can guide us to effective stress management by communicating our problems with others.

Share your problems with friends or other non-work colleagues

Yallom (1970), an influential psychoanalyst, identified that sharing problems with others, even if they don't help us solve any problems, helps us feel like we're not alone. We can realise that others have faced similar problems, people can empathise with us and take our side and, in effect, validate our stressful experience. Sometimes people might use phrases like 'I know what you mean', 'that happened to me' or 'that must have upset you'. Yallom calls this effect **'universality'** because we realise we share similar feelings with others – it's not just us! This is a good approach when stressed by things you can't easily change, such as your assignment deadlines or practice setting.

Explain your problems to colleagues

This is a different approach to stress because, by explaining the cause of your stress to colleagues, you are seeking to solve a problem or look for help in managing the problem better. There is a goal involved here: you are not just 'offloading' on to others as in the above example.

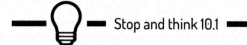

Stop and think 10.1

Why do you think it is better to explain a problem to colleagues rather than 'offload' your feelings?

Some of the answers you may have thought about can be identified in the next paragraph.

We can see that simply 'offloading' onto colleagues would be sharing a problem that they also experience and possibly already have an opinion about. Yes, they may agree with us, but work colleagues are in the same situation as us and we will not get that sense of 'universalism' from people who are 'in the same boat'. However, if we are seeking to solve a problem, work colleagues are often in the best position to help as they know the situation and the options available. Problem-solving is even more effective if we can include a line manager, clinical supervisor or personal tutor who is in a position to make any necessary changes. Be aware also that we can make ourselves more stressed by thinking stressfully.

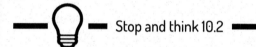

Stop and think 10.2

Have a look at Tables 7.1 and 7.2 on dysfunctional and unhelpful thinking in Chapter 7. Do you recognise any of the unhelpful thinking styles? Beware the student's favourite unhelpful thought, 'It's not fair!'

Writing in clinical practice

Nurses are required to keep written records in relation to care (NMC, 2018b) in their workplace and students need to develop these skills to a professional standard in order to qualify for registration. Student nurses are often all too aware that academic writing is part of the assessment process in training, and qualified practitioners will also have to write academic essays to acquire post-registration qualification and demonstrate continuing professional development. We will look firstly at writing in the practice setting.

Documenting practice: enhancing care and safeguarding patients

See Box 10.1, which lists the standards for record-keeping according to the NMC *Code* (NMC, 2018b).

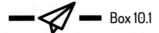 Box 10.1

NMC standards for record-keeping

- Complete records at the time or as soon as possible after an event; if the notes are written some time after an event, record this in the notes.
- Identify any risks or problems that have arisen and the steps taken to deal with them, so that colleagues who use the records have all the information they need.
- Complete records accurately and without any falsification, taking immediate and appropriate action if you become aware that someone has not kept to these requirements.
- Attribute any entries you make in any paper or electronic records to yourself, making sure they are clearly written, dated and timed, and do not include unnecessary abbreviations, jargon or speculation.
- Take all steps to make sure that records are kept securely.
- Collect, treat and store all data and research findings appropriately.

(NMC, 2018b:11)

Nursing care plans should be used to facilitate, record and measure care (Ballantyne, 2016). Care plans and patient records are regarded as legal documents which can be used as evidence in a court of law. Therefore it is vital that nurses record data accurately, realistically and without prejudice and bias. It is important that entries on patient records are worded in such a way as to convey information as objective and observable facts, and that these facts are true, supportable and include all important details and do not exclude important and relevant details. The wording and style of writing is important to reflect the elements of record-keeping outlined below.

Objectivity

Data that is objective is free from bias and assumptions. The only element of subjectivity may be the professional opinion of the practitioner who is, by virtue of their skills and knowledge, able to make a degree of professional judgement equal to their training and experience. Data also should be free from moral judgement based on values and norms of the practitioner and free from stigma or prejudice.

Data that is observable and supportable

Data entered into patient records or care plans need to describe measurable and observable behaviour and facts. The nurse needs to be able to account objectively for the data on what they have observed. Data should only be based on evidence the nurse can be accountable for. This therefore rules out the nurse's opinion (which is outside professional judgement) or assumptions. A nurse can describe a patient as having 'appeared upset', but should not simply say 'the patient was upset'. If a patient says they are upset, the appropriate objective recording of this would be 'the patient reported being upset'.

Relevance

Recorded data should be clearly related to aspects of the patient's care. If a specific nursing model or approach is used, nursing observations may be structured according to the elements of the model. For instance, in Roper's model of Activities of Daily Living (ADL) (Holland et al., 2008), observations will reflect an ADL. Sometimes entries are made that relate to ADLs but are not relevant to care. For instance, the often overused 'slept well' may not have anything to do with a person's reasons for needing care. Nurses still record this, however, although it is not usually supportable information, unless the nurse sat by the bedside and observed the patient snoring happily all night!

Entries for patient records should aid the evaluation aspect of the nursing process and record whether interventions were carried out and how they were carried out. Care plan entries should clearly state specific care instructions which include the rationale for interventions and the aims or goals. Look at Tables 10.1 and 10.2 for examples of good practice and poor practice in record-keeping.

Table 10.1 Care plan and notes for patient X

Rationale (assessed need)	Aim (plan)	Action (intervention)	Evaluation	Notes
Patient demonstrates 24-hour over-activity, has difficulty getting to sleep and maintaining sleep for more than 2 hours during the night.	For the patient to establish a stable sleep pattern	1 To encourage patient to adhere to planned sleep/wake regime, 11 pm–6 am rest period 2-10. [*] 11 To monitor patient's periods of restfulness in bed	1 Record observed sleep pattern in sleep diary 2 Obtain patient's report of sleep pattern 3 Review sleep plan weekly	Day 1: 1 Patient reminded of sleep plan 3 times between 11 pm and 11.30 pm. 2-10. [*] 11 Patient lay on bed in day clothes until 12 pm. Remained until 2.30 am. Active in ward till 4 am, then returned to bed and appeared to sleep until 5.30 am. Active on ward to present (7 am). Patient reported having slept 'most of the night'.

* Details omitted in this example for brevity.

Table 10.2   Care plan and notes for patient Y

Rationale (assessed need)	Aim (plan)	Action (intervention)	Evaluation	Notes
Patient suffers from bipolar disorder, in manic phase	Patient to establish normal sleep pattern	1 Encourage patient to get to bed at 11 pm and stay in bed till 6 am 2–10. [*] 11 Observe sleep pattern	1 Complete sleep diary 2 Review diary in 1 week	Day 1: Patient went to bed late evening Got up once during night, otherwise slept well

* Details omitted in this example for brevity.

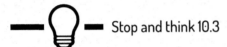 Stop and think 10.3

Looking at the care plan examples in Tables 10.1 and 10.2, can you identify:

1   Words that describe observable data
2   Words or phrases that describe value judgements or assumptions
3   Words that give specific and relevant instructions
4   Words or phrases that give vague instructions or information
5   Words or phrases that are not relevant or are inaccurate.

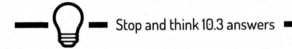 Stop and think 10.3 answers

1   Words that describe observable data:

'restfulness', '3 times', 'active', 'lay on bed', 'appeared to sleep' and all specific timed events;

2   Words or phrases that describe value judgements or assumptions:

'normal sleep pattern'   need to establish what is 'normal' for this patient when well

'patient suffers from bipolar disorder, in manic phase'   assumes over-activity is due to diagnosis, also assumes patient 'suffers' because of the diagnosis

'slept well'   assumes that the patient actually slept and this was good quality sleep; this is not observable;

3   Words that give specific and relevant instructions or information:

all data in Table 10.1

time of sleep plan as an action and 'review diary in one week', in Table 10.2;

4   Words or phrases that give vague instructions:

most of Table 10.2, except as above

Table 10.1 contains some necessarily vague instructions that are open to nursing judgement, such as 'stable', 'restfulness', 'encourage', 'monitor', 'reminded' and 'active';

5   Words or phrases that are not relevant or are inaccurate:

'patient suffers from bipolar disorder'   the patient's diagnosis is irrelevant; their behaviour (over-activity) is relevant to the care need (sleep)

'observe sleep pattern'   how will this be observed and recorded?

'review diary' (Table 10.2)   this is not supported by a clear aim except a 'normal' sleep pattern; Table 10.1, at least, relies on something measurable – a 'stable' sleep pattern (i.e. regular, consistent).

Format of information

Records can be presented in a number of formats, including written records, electronic records or using a visual image. Different formats work for different types of information. The selection of the format will often depend on the intended purpose and audience involved. The following section will discuss the collection and use of different types and formats of information in more depth.

Written record

It is common for nursing notes and patient records to be handwritten or typed. The use of a model or framework for assessment can reduce the amount of time required to undertake the process and can ensure consistency of assessment and standardised documentation for every patient. In most instances, handwritten information is completed on standardised pro-forma templates which the organisation applies to all patients.

Nursing records of daily care are often written in free text and may be very subjective. The use of free text can often lead to the use of jargon and abbreviations which only the nurse making the entry may understand. This may lead to misunderstandings between staff regarding recording of events or the care delivered.

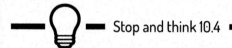

Stop and think 10.4

Consider the abbreviations you have come across in practice. Do you know what they all mean and what impact do you think the use of abbreviations in a patient's notes may have?

Nurses use a lot of abbreviations when handing over and discussing care and in their documentation but it is important that records are clear and transparent in both their legibility and translation. There are hundreds of abbreviations used in healthcare. Acceptable ones may include C&R (control and restraint), ED (emergency department), COPD (chronic obstructive pulmonary disease), CVA (cardiovascular accident) and DDA (Disability Discrimination Act). Many organisations produce a glossary of acceptable abbreviations for that specific workplace. It is vital that health professionals do not invent their own abbreviations which may cause confusion in patient records or prescriptions, for instance. If you have any doubts about your interpretation of an abbreviation you should check it to maintain safe and effective care.

Handwriting is often very difficult to read and if the information is unclear then it is easy to see how errors may occur. Inferences are drawn by the reader about what the writer meant. The person who has written the information may have a different understanding of the information than the person reading it.

Misinterpretations of information account for many clinical errors. According to the National Patient Safety Agency (2018) there were 204,162 medication errors reported in 2017. Year on year, approximately 30% of such errors are attributable to prescribing errors, with many due to the prescription being unclear.

Electronic records

The use of information technology in healthcare means that many forms of communication are now completed electronically. In the NHS there are many examples of electronic systems for data collection and information storage, formats for which are being updated frequently.

Electronic information may be sent in written format or by pro-forma completed online using a set of pre-existing criteria. A typical example of this is an electronic incident reporting system. Usually, the incident report number is generated by the system automatically and a series of pre-set criteria are utilised by the person reporting the incident to outline the type of incident, date, time and details. It could be compared with using an online booking system for an airline. The system is set up to offer choices of pre-set information and the user clicks on the appropriate choice and the system then records that choice. Electronic systems may allow a combination of pre-set information and free text, as could an incident reporting system.

Care planning systems are also available in practice which use set frameworks to allow the nurse to assess a patient, plan and record care. Some systems have pre-set criteria which assist the nurse in defining the process required for assessing a specific patient, but the disadvantage may be that they do not always meet the needs of individual patients. Other systems may be more flexible and allow free text input which ensures the nurse can meet the needs of the individual patient.

Visual image records

Visual images are often useful in documenting specific care of patients. Pictures can represent the stages of wound healing which provide more accurate information than the written word. This is particularly useful if a patient's care is being delivered by a range of people and over a prolonged period of time as it allows them to see the difference between the stages of wound healing without having seen the actual wound.

Images can also be stored to represent cases or specific diseases which help us to develop our knowledge and understanding in relation to a specific subject. The use of visual images often helps to illustrate a subject or a point of view in a way that words simply could not. Examples include the use of diagrams to represent family trees in a patient's record or diagrams of the body to document the distribution of a patient's injuries.

The same rules apply to written, electronic and visual methods of communicating patient care: they need to be observable, objective and relevant.

Academic writing: how to get your message across

Writing an essay is an essential skill for nursing students as it constitutes a high proportion of the material by which you will be assessed. The main reason for examining nurses by their written work is to have evidence of the student's ability to understand the theory behind practice, to demonstrate their ability to evaluate and critically analyse theoretical evidence and to demonstrate a practical ability to make links between theory and practice. Hence many marked assignments ask students to evaluate or critically analyse some aspect of theory and apply it to a practice situation. Most written assignments in nursing are likely to take this form in one way or another. So, while whole books and courses can be dedicated to improving student writing skills, this section will focus specifically on aiding you to identify what exactly is being asked of you in an assignment, and how to answer that question so you can demonstrate that you have attained the right level of understanding and knowledge.

Identifying what is being asked of you

Assignment writers need to set a task that gives a fair opportunity for the student to demonstrate key learning outcomes on specified theory-to-practice themes. These key learning outcomes guide the marking process and are easy to spot in the marking criteria and assignment brief. They use specific words, called **descriptors** in educational language, and which are always verbs or adverbs (words that describe actions or words that describe *how* an action is performed), in the assignment and criteria sentences. See below:

Descriptors: they tell you what to do, and how to do it.

Describe a nursing model and *critically discuss* its use in a practice setting.

The two verb descriptors in this example are *describe* and *discuss*. The sentence also tells you *how* to perform one of those tasks with the adverb descriptor *critically*.

Next, the assignment will tell you what the topic is. This is what you are expected to talk about. In the above example, the topic is *a nursing model*.

The final element of an assignment like this is the context, and in nursing this is invariably some form of nursing practice context – clinical, managerial or research-based.

In our example, the context is *a practice setting*, so we can take it that this means a clinical setting, although there is no reason in this case why we couldn't also look at the impact of a model on the care management element of practice.

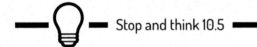 Stop and think 10.5

Look at the assignment examples below and identify:

a   What the student is being asked to do (the verb descriptors)
b   How the student is to do it (the adverb descriptors)
c   The topic the student should address
d   The context in which the student should address the topic.

Examples:

1   Choose a chronic illness and describe and discuss three health promotion strategies that enable patients to adopt self-care to better manage their condition.
2   Critically evaluate any nursing intervention of your choice in relation to improving patient safety in the hospital setting.
3   Identify a specific health need commonly encountered in community nursing; describe and critically evaluate the key service provision resources provided to meet that need.
4   Identify and describe a reflective model and critically analyse its effectiveness in aiding an aspect of professional development.

How did you do?
Answers:

1
   a   Descriptors: describe, discuss
   b   Adverb descriptors: no adverb descriptors given
   c   The topic: three health promotion strategies (of your choice)
   d   The context: patient self-care

2
  a   Descriptor: evaluate
  b   Adverb descriptor: critically
  c   The topic: improving patient safety
  d   The context: a hospital setting (of your choice)

3
  a   Descriptors: identify, describe, evaluate
  b   Adverb descriptor: critically
  c   The topic: service provision resources
  d   The context: a common community health need (of your choice)

4
  a   Descriptors: identify, describe, analyse
  b   Adverb descriptor: critically
  c   The topic: a reflective model (of your choice)
  d   The context: one aspect of professional development (of your choice)

Sometimes descriptors, topics and contexts can be obscured in the sentence construction. It can help in such circumstances to rewrite the sentence yourself to make it clearer. The example in Box 10.2 identifies the key elements of a complex question, which aids its simplification.

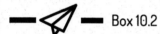 **Box 10.2**

Assignment task

Here's the assignment: 'Using a patient or client you have cared for in practice, describe one aspect of care and discuss and critically analyse the evidence underpinning the nursing care given. Discuss how well the care given complied with the need to apply evidence-based practice in nursing care.'

This can be re-worded for clarity, as in Box 10.3.

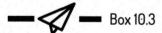 **Box 10.3**

Rewritten version

Here's the rewritten version: 'Using a case study and one aspect of care, discuss and critically analyse evidence which supports the care given. Discuss how well it complied with evidence-based nursing practice.'

Notice that the descriptors (underlined) and the topics to be covered are still there.

The descriptors, topic and context also tell us what not to do. If the words *describe*, *list* and *identify* are not there, it can be assumed that lengthy descriptions of, say, Roper's model or diabetes, are not necessary. We can save words and get on with *discussing* or *critically analysing* because that is where the marks will be offered.

Structuring your answer: how to write an essay

An essay is a story but in a different form to a fictional account. Like a story it has a beginning, a middle and an end. The example below will help you 'tell your story' for most essays in nursing.

Beginning: the introduction

Say what you are going to talk about, and say why the topic is important (to healthcare). And that's it! There is no need to go on at this point. Most students waste loads of word space here. It is unnecessary.

Middle: your discussion/critique/evaluation

You don't need to repeat what you have already said in the introduction. Get on with addressing the descriptors in the assignment guidelines or question. See some examples below:

a   *Describe* your topic and the context in which it takes place.

Roper's model (Roper et al., 1981) is ... .

Patient X was a 43-year-old man with type 2 diabetes and needed ... .

b   *Discuss* the relevance/importance of the patient's needs to the topic.

Patient X's main need appeared to be best met by the Y aspect of the model because ... .

c   *Evaluate* the effectiveness of the topic in the context of care.

Roper's model helped nurses identify and meet the patient's needs; however, Orem's self-care model may have been more useful in identifying the patient's self-care abilities, such as ... .

d   *Critically analyse*: use the material you have described, discussed and evaluated to then explain why you think the situation was as it was. You can also suggest what could improve the situation.

Roper's model was probably used in this case because the nurses were familiar with ... . Lack of skills development may have limited staff members' flexibility of model use and so ... .

This section of the essay should contain all the key evidence that demonstrates your knowledge, understanding and ability to discuss, evaluate and critically analyse the topic in the specific context.

The end: your conclusion or summary

The golden rule with your conclusion is not to introduce new material. However, the section is often a student's saviour because, if there hasn't been much critical analysis or evaluation before, here is the last chance to demonstrate these skills. This section should aim to remind the reader what the 'argument' has been, and a simple sentence in the conclusion can do this. For example:

> Therefore, it could be argued that adoption of one model on a ward can limit flexibility in meeting the wider holistic needs of some patients.

A good summary shows the reader that you understand the implications of what you have detailed previously. So, *don't* repeat yourself, but *do* sum up your take-home message in one or two sentences in this section.

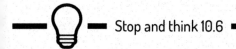

Look up some examples of past exam papers or assignments in your academic institution and try the following.

1   Identify the descriptors, topic(s) and contexts that are required.
2   Rewrite long or complex assignment briefs into your own questions. Try to be as succinct and clear as possible without changing the task.
3   Write a very brief outline consisting only of headings and sub-headings that you might use for such an assignment, starting with the main headings introduction, discussion and conclusion.

Surviving presentations

Making a presentation to colleagues or fellow students or for a formal assignment is usually seen by students as very stressful and challenging. Few of us feel comfortable speaking formally to an audience, even if they are friends. Student nurses have to demonstrate their ability to disseminate knowledge and provide learning to others, so it is an important communication skill that needs to be developed. The good thing is, once you have done a few presentations on the course, you will feel much more confident when doing them professionally. We all need to be able to develop skills in disseminating good practice to our colleagues as a requirement of the NMC *Code* (NMC, 2018b). We may also be required to deliver educational or health promotional material to students, patients or carers, for example on sexual health or smoking cessation in schools or primary care, or stress management in psychiatric settings. So, it is a skill that will prepare you for practice!

The key enemy to a good presentation is nerves! If you are not used to speaking in public, the very act of standing in front of an audience is a challenge in itself. The best way to reduce this problem is practice! Practise in front of your friends, family or colleagues at work, anywhere and everywhere. This is a theory- and practice-based technique linked to behavioural principles: the more we expose ourselves to feared stimuli and survive without harm, the more our nervous reactions will reduce.

Knowledge link See Chapter 7 on behavioural principles for reassurance on this fact. You can also engage in positive and realistic thinking (again, see Chapter 7).

Remind yourself that you will not die, the audience will not hate you and will probably be helpful and empathetic, that what you have to say is important or interesting (all good cognitive behavioural techniques) and that it will be a good step to developing your presentation skills so that next time you will be even better at it!

Organisation and planning

Poor planning and organisation can reduce the success of a presentation. A useful checklist will help you focus your planning for a streamlined presentation. This takes us through *who, what, where, when, how* and *why*.

Who will be your audience? During nurse training it will be either fellow students and your tutor or nursing colleagues on your practice placement. Qualified nurses may be presenting to nursing or multi-disciplinary clinical colleagues in their workplace or to patient groups or students. The key factor is gauging what the audience already knows and how to pitch your descriptive material in the presentation; not over their heads but don't waste time explaining the obvious.

What is your topic? The key element is to ensure you are familiar with the subject or at least plan the presentation to highlight the key areas. In structuring a presentation, keep the subject matter relevant and work towards the 'take-home message'. A tip that might help is to plan the presentation from the bottom up; identify the point you are aiming for and work backwards from there. Ask yourself, what does the audience need to know in order to fully understand my key point?

Where are you presenting? Check out the environment, the equipment and where you will stand or sit. Will you be interrupted? Will there be noise? How can you limit these potential problems? Try to 'take control' of the environment. Don't just rely on someone else to do it. Move furniture, arrange your notes and close windows or curtains. Do whatever it takes to take control.

How long have you got? A short presentation means clear and relevant facts only, with bullet points, a short introduction and getting straight to the point. Longer presentations mean you can introduce a bit more detail and even entertain your audience! Tell a few anecdotes that relate to the subject! Keep your audience interested by switching focus.

Keep it interesting! If you are using something like Microsoft PowerPoint, avoid putting too many words on each slide. Use bullet points only, supported by a picture or diagram – something entertaining or a relevant graph. Put only five or six points on each slide and use the slide as your notes or prompt sheet. It saves having notes in your hands and getting lost!

Why are you making this presentation? Focus on the main aim of the presentation. Is it to educate practitioners or students? Is it to pass a marked assessment? Is it to practise giving presentations? Is it to present group work or study material? Ask yourself: what is it I want to achieve? If it is a marked assessment, plan your presentation around the marking criteria. If it is to impart knowledge, focus on the key points you want the audience to appreciate and remember. Planning towards an identified goal again is helped by bottom-up planning. Work from the goal back to the method of achieving it.

Here's a reminder of key points for surviving presentations:

- think positively and realistically
- know your topic
- plan
- identify your goals
- take control.

Conclusion

This chapter has focused on some core professional skills needed particularly for nursing care management and personal and professional development. Writing skills and record-keeping are needed to communicate patient care needs clearly to our colleagues, using care plans and patient records. We also need good writing skills in order to disseminate ideas in evidence-based practice to justify our care and demonstrate our professional development. As a student you will need to do this through writing formal assignments during your training. As a qualified nurse you will need to demonstrate continuing professional development through post-registration training and course work, and to support your professional role in disseminating good practice to fellow professionals. We also need formal verbal skills to disseminate learning and evidence-based practice to our colleagues through making presentations. As nurses, we may also use presentation skills to deliver health promotion to patients and the general public. It may be the case that student nurses think that academic writing and presenting is not important to nursing after qualification; that these skills are only required in order to get through the pre-registration course. However, as has been highlighted, these skills are required of a qualified nurse to meet the demands of the NMC *Code* (NMC, 2018b) and to practise as a competent nurse.

FURTHER READING

Murray, N. and Hughes, G. (2008) *Writing Up Your University Assignments and Research Projects*. Maidenhead, McGraw-Hill Education.

NMC (2018) *Realising Professionalism: Standards for Education and Training. Part 1: Standards Framework for Nursing and Midwifery Education*. London, Nursing and Midwifery Council.

REFERENCES

Ballantyne, H. (2016) Developing nursing care plans. *Nursing Standard*, 30(26), 51–57.

Goleman, D. (2004) *What Makes a Leader?* Harvard Business Review. https://cdn.ymaws.com/aect.site-ym.com/resource/dynamic/forums/20130118_183018_26306.pdf.

Holland, K., Jenkins, J., Solomon, J. and Whittam, S. (2008) *Applying the Roper, Logan and Tierney Model in Practice* (2nd edn). Edinburgh, Churchill Livingstone.

Lauder, W., Roxburgh, M., Holland, K., Johnson, M., Watson, W., Porter, M., Topping, K. and Behr, A. (2008) *Nursing and Midwifery in Scotland: Being Fit for Practice*. Dundee, University of Dundee.

Mackintosh, C. (2006) Caring: the socialisation of pre-registration student nurses: a longitudinal qualitative descriptive study. *International Journal of Nursing Studies*, 43, 953–962.

Murray, K. (2014) *Building Resilience in Midwifery and Nursing Staff*. Blog/BMJ Nursing. https://blogs.bmj.com/ebn/2014/03/31/building-resilience-in-midwifery-and-nursing-staff/.

National Patient Safety Agency (2018) *National Patient Safety Incident Reports: 26 September 2018*. London, NHS Improvement.

NMC (2018a) *Part 1: Standards Framework for Nursing and Midwifery Education*. www.nmc.org.uk/globalassets/sitedocuments/education-standards/education-framework.pdf

NMC (2018b) *The Code: Professional Standards of Practice and Behaviour for Nurses, Midwives and Nursing Associates*. www.nmc.org.uk/standards/code/.

Pulido-Martos, M., Augusto-Landa, J.M. and Lopez-Zafra, E. (2012) Sources of stress in nursing students: a systematic review of quantitative studies. *International Nursing Review*, 59, 15–25.

Thomson, R., Docherty, A. and Duffy, R. (2017) Nursing students' experiences of mentorship in their final placement. *British Journal of Nursing*, 26(9), 514–521.

Yallom, D. (1970) *The Theory & Practice of Group Psychotherapy*. New York, Basic Books.

PART III
ADVANCING APPLICATION OF COMMUNICATION SKILLS

Preface to Part 3

The final part of this book addresses communication and interpersonal skills through application in specific clinical scenarios. While the material in this book does not aim to separate different fields of care, this part acknowledges that different clinical areas demand specific skills in interpersonal communication.

One chapter in this section therefore looks specifically at short-term and immediate care (Chapter 11). This could be acute psychiatric settings or emergency and acute care departments. The skills, however, can apply to any setting where immediate care is required. Another chapter (Chapter 12) will examine the other end of the spectrum of care by focusing on long-term and chronic care settings. This acknowledges that nurse–patient relationships can be enduring and have specific health goals such as developing self-management. We also address the specific needs of children and young people and the communication skills that need to be deployed at different developmental levels (Chapter 13). This part also addresses care for those with cognitive impairments that limit their ability to communicate (Chapter 14). Again, the nurse is challenged to be adaptive, supporting and understanding, and to maintain a non-judgemental approach to the interpersonal relationship. We return to examine health promotion in more detail, examining more specific and sometimes specialist skills that, regardless of field of care, we can all adopt for non-specialist interventions (Chapter 15). Finally, we extend the communication skills to your management and how you can deploy a range of communication approaches to aid your own professional development (Chapter 16).

All these skills will be with you for the duration of your career, and beyond, and we hope you will continue to develop all the skills you have been exposed to in this book and so deliver excellent care to your patients.

ELEVEN
COMMUNICATING IN IMMEDIATE AND SHORT-TERM CARE SITUATIONS

ANNE-MARIE BORNEUF AND JACQUI GLADWIN

THIS CHAPTER WILL HELP YOU TO ACHIEVE
COMPETENCIES IN:

- Managing and diffusing challenging situations
- Communicating safely and effectively
- Being proactive and creative in enhancing communication
- Using appropriate and relevant communication skills to deal with challenging circumstances
- Selecting and applying strategies and techniques for conflict resolution
- Working confidently as part of the team and as leader of the team

Introduction

Managing acutely ill or injured patients in an acute care setting places particular demands on the therapeutic nurse–patient relationship and calls for higher-order communication skills. Variables that pose particular challenges include a high turnover of patients and the potential for the rapid deterioration of the patient's condition. We can add to these challenges, with anxiety levels of staff, patients and their family members adding tension as, indeed, do sudden alterations in the dynamics of the care team due to the number of patients requiring specialist care at a moment's notice. The diverse nature of the patient population also requires nurses to tailor their communication styles moment by moment to achieve effective and safe care delivery for all patients.

This chapter will address specific communication challenges when responding to acute care needs. In any acute event, the nursing management of patients in acute pain or who are psychologically disturbed, emotionally distressed, angry or fearful relies on confident communication and self-management skills. In the emergency care setting, for example, team members need to co-ordinate their actions, follow set protocols and transfer information to other health professionals. In this chapter we will demonstrate some of the specific communication approaches in application and challenge you to apply knowledge covered in earlier chapters to your field of care.

The challenges of communication in diverse acute care settings

Acute care settings are often fast-paced or intense environments. They include the emergency department (or accident and emergency), intensive care, psychiatric intensive care units (PICU), neonatal intensive care and intensive care units (NICU and ICU) and high-dependency as well as medical assessment units (MAU). However, nurses of all fields are likely to need to respond to acute care needs, which may occur in the community or care home. It is important to have the skills and knowledge to respond to acute and short-term care needs. While much of this chapter focuses on typical acute care settings, the skills and understanding are relevant to all fields of nursing.

Acute care settings can be difficult places to work. They deal with a range of patients of diverse backgrounds and cultures, different ages, including children, and a variety of acute physical or mental health conditions. Teams working in this environment will be made up of different professionals who need to communicate effectively in order to manage the volume of activity in the department and ensure the safety of patients and staff. The nature of acute settings means that there will be a requirement to communicate across professions and agencies both within healthcare and outside it.

Patients who are admitted to acute care environments are often acutely or even critically ill, in pain, anxious, frightened and often disorientated. They may have relatives in attendance who are also anxious and frightened. There will be patients with a range of problems, both minor and major, and each will have different communication needs. A key priority for all will be provision of and access to information and a calm reassuring approach from the nurse providing the care.

With the exception of intensive care units, most acute care settings are noisy and busy areas. The turnover and volume of patients can be high, coupled with the frequent interruption of emergency patient situations which need to be dealt with quickly. This can be extremely frightening for patients and their families, especially if they have limited experience of this type of environment. It can also be frightening for students who have not been exposed to patients with traumatic injuries or displaying psychotic symptoms.

Pierre et al. (2007) identify the following reasons why communication is so complex in acute care:

- uncertainty
- information overload
- time pressures
- risk
- multiple people involved
- multiple goals and priorities.

The unique nature of acute care environments is such that all the above factors combine to create challenging situations. Therefore, a nurse needs to possess effective communication skills which can be easily adapted and flexible enough to cope with the fast pace and diverse group of people they will come into contact with.

Managing patients who have difficulties communicating is always challenging for nurses but even more so when acute care is needed. Acutely ill patients often have complex needs and those who have been admitted to hospital as an emergency will need to be assessed and prioritised effectively and quickly in order to ensure that their needs are met. Problems with language are often increased, as there may not be easy access to interpreters, especially outside normal hours, and patients are too distressed to express themselves clearly or take in verbal information.

Patients with a learning disability or a mental health problem may often become very agitated and distressed in an acute environment. They can often become more difficult to manage or communicate with, and the nurse must identify their needs quickly to reduce the patient's anxiety and fear and promote effective communication between themselves, the patient and the carers or family.

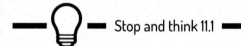 Stop and think 11.1

Identify and list some situations where communication has been a challenge in an acute care event. Write down in your reflective diary what made these situations challenging.

Priorities for high-risk patients

In order to assess patients quickly and prioritise care, nurses can enhance their communication skills by following procedures. For example, in EDs and acute admission units, nurses often use a model of triage to identify and rule out any life-threatening problems. Triage models such as Manchester Triage (Manchester Triage Group, 2013) incorporate a system of flow charts relating to specific conditions. The nurse then assesses the patient using the flow chart to establish their priority for treatment. If the patient is suffering from a life-threatening or high-risk condition, communication with the patient may not be possible and the nurse will usually identify the level of priority from the presenting physiological or behavioural signs.

For patients presenting with lower-risk conditions the nurse can focus their communication approach to assess the patient more fully and ask questions to confirm that they do not require immediate treatment. For psychiatric states, for instance, the assessment will address the patient's risk of harm to self and others. For a thorough assessment, this demands specialist interviewing skills but in the first instance risk can be ascertained by sensitive questioning and listening, guided by the use of risk-assessment tools. The importance of effective history-taking should not be underestimated. Diagnosis is primarily made on the history a patient provides and so effective communication skills are essential to obtain a full and detailed history.

Impaired ability to communicate

Patients with acute conditions often have impaired ability to communicate. This may be temporary or permanent. A patient who has had an acute stroke may suffer acute **dysphasia**, and patients with traumatic injuries may have reduced consciousness or damage to their hearing or speech functions.

The NMC (2018) clearly identifies, in the *Code*, that a nurse has a role to practise as an effective communicator for patients and as such must find ways to represent their views even if they have impaired communication:

> take reasonable steps to meet people's language and communication needs, providing, wherever possible, assistance to those who need help to communicate their own or other people's needs.
>
> (NMC, 2018:9)

The challenge for nurses in this environment will often be that they have limited knowledge of the patient and therefore may not be able to understand the subtle forms of communication the patient may use. Family members may be vital in interpreting a patient's efforts to communicate and nurses must try to establish some form of communication with patients as early as possible. This concept is supported by Blackburn et al. (2019) who identify the importance of communication for reducing anxieties and improving the overall experience of acute care, and ensuring patients and families are fully involved in their care.

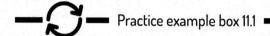 Practice example box 11.1

Communicating with a patient who has had a stroke

Mr Jones, a 35-year-old man, is admitted to the ED following a stroke, is ventilated and mildly sedated and being nursed in an intensive care unit. He is able to communicate with staff and family using his eyes and his hands only.

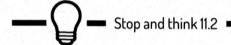 Stop and think 11.2

Read Practice example box 11.1. What will the challenges be for ensuring that Mr Jones has his communication needs met and how might the nurse support and develop his limited ability to communicate?

Possible answer: touch, eye contact, facial expressions, simple gestures and non-verbal responding (tapping, blinking, etc.) to closed questions (requiring only yes/no answers). Ask family members to interpret the patient's gestures as they know him best. For simple communication, picture boards can be used to indicate choices.

Intoxication

A significant challenge in acute areas is patients or their relatives who are intoxicated with alcohol or drugs. Alcohol-related attendances to EDs can range from 12% to as high as 70% of all attendances at weekends (Parkinson et al., 2016).

Intoxication in patients in whatever form causes some degree of cerebral impairment (Brown and Cadogan, 2016), which may lead to an acute confusional state or an impaired ability to communicate or process information effectively. It is important to be clear about whether the person is intoxicated with recreational substances or has a medical condition. Possible causes of confusion and impaired functioning include metabolic disorders such as diabetes or hypoxia, or congenital or pathological causes such as learning disability, dementia or psychosis.

Intoxicated patients or relatives, if not at risk, are thankfully most likely to become sleepy because of the sedating effect of alcohol and common street drugs. Management of service users when they are in a talkative or agitated state demands assertive management and a **closing down** approach. This is the use of short answers, closed questions and even ignoring irrelevant chatter or behaviour. Be careful not to encourage further unhelpful behaviour by responding to chatter or inappropriate behaviour if you have other care priorities. See Practice example box 11.2.

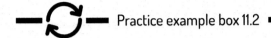 Practice example box 11.2

Using a closing down approach

A highly overactive patient arrived on a psychiatric intensive care unit with very fast speech (pressure of speech) and high distractibility. He would not sit down but paced the room and frequently interrupted the nurse with irrelevant questions as she was attempting to take a brief history. The nurse allowed the patient to pace the room and found that by ignoring the questions and keeping to closed questions herself, the history was taken adequately for his short-term care.

Knowledge link Look back to Chapter 7 on operant conditioning, which shows how rewarding or ignoring certain behaviour can increase or diminish it.

Aggression

Patients or relatives who are intoxicated, frightened or confused may be aggressive towards the staff. The acute care environment can often precipitate or escalate aggression in individuals and the nurse should be aware of the potential for aggression in a range of patients. EDs can often appear hostile and threatening to patients and relatives who may be in an emotionally charged state (Dolan and Holt, 2013). Acute or sudden illness will often be accompanied by great anxiety and fear for both patient and family. Nurses can use the environment and their communication skills to diffuse aggression through giving attention, information and reassurance and by removing the source of annoyance from the person – or the other way around! During any acute care episode be aware of the challenges the environment bring to situations and have a risk-aware approach to maintaining their own and others' safety. For example, ensure that you are always aware of where the exit route is, and make sure the patient is never between you and the door. Avoid getting backed into areas without an exit and make sure you don't have equipment such as scissors or stethoscopes sticking out of your pockets or around your neck. Be aware of potential weapons and be alert to any patients or relatives who behave oddly or have previous history of violence against staff. Being aware and prepared are the greatest tools a nurse has in this area of work when it comes to minimising the risk of harm.

Knowledge link Chapter 8 gives specific details on de-escalation techniques and managing aggression.

Multi-disciplinary communication

There is often a need to communicate with other professionals in an acute setting. The handover of patients between professionals is extremely important. Patients may arrive by ambulance or with the police, social services, etc. The nurse's role is to ensure an effective handover from the professional accompanying the patient. Equally, the nurse must then provide an effective handover of care from either the ED or the ward to theatre, or the intensive care unit. The acute nature of the area will often mean that the patient has undergone a substantial amount of assessment, investigation and treatment. This care should be recorded accurately and then communicated to the receiving team.

Confidentiality

In situations where there is the possibility that patient confidentiality may have to be breached because of the need for child protection or because a crime has been committed, the nurse must ensure that all communications are recorded. If a nurse has to give evidence in a court of law then they cannot claim privilege due to their professional position (Dolan and Holt, 2013).

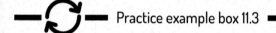 Practice example box 11.3

Limits of confidentiality

A man with a disulfiram implant (a medication designed to react negatively with alcohol) was admitted through ED with a severe reaction to alcohol, including very high blood pressure. He had driven himself to the ED the previous evening and on discharge in the morning intended to drive home. He was advised that he was still intoxicated but he insisted on getting into his car and driving away. The nurses contacted the police and reported his actions. He was stopped, breathalysed and arrested for drink-driving.

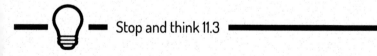 Stop and think 11.3

In Practice example box 11.3 how would the nurses justify breaching confidentiality in this case by revealing to the police that this man was still under the influence of alcohol? Can you find the relevant parts in the NMC *Code* (NMC, 2018), and where should the nurses record their actions?

(Continued)

Answer: the NMC *Code* tells you to:

- Act without delay if you believe that there is a risk to patient safety or public protection
- Share information if you believe someone may be at risk of harm, in line with the laws relating to disclosure of information.

(NMC, 2018)

The nurses' actions should be recorded factually in the patient's notes (especially that he was advised not to drive) and, in accordance with many NHS Trust policies, also reported on an incident form.

Developing communication skills

This section will address the communication skills required by nurses working in acute care areas when managing a range of patient issues. There are a range of situations that present as communication complexities and nurses may need to adapt their communication skills to be effective. Experiencing these situations helps to develop our abilities and ensure we communicate effectively for future challenges that we will face in this discipline.

Case management

Research has illustrated that interruptive communication seems to dominate in high-stress medical environments (Alvarez and Coiera, 2005). Reflect on the last time a patient or relative asked you a question or a query: how many times have you said 'I'll get back to you in a minute!' because you are busy dealing with a previous enquiry. Interruptions take place within the workplace all the time. Take a look at Practice example box 11.4.

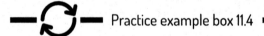 Practice example box 11.4

Prioritising needs

Mr Smith, 89, is brought to the ED by ambulance from a nursing home. He is dehydrated and has a large pressure ulcer on his sacrum. He is disorientated and has a left-sided weakness due to a previous stroke. The paramedic hands the patient over but a carer has not escorted him from the nursing home. The patient is extremely distressed and frightened. Mr Smith's daughter arrives and is very angry about the care her father has received at the nursing home. She is also upset that he is in the ED and has not been admitted straight to a ward. She is confrontational and clearly distressed.

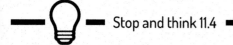 Stop and think 11.4

Outline how you may deal with the situation in Practice example box 11.4 and identify the skills required for effective communication in this scenario. Clues are given in the text below!

As indicated earlier in this chapter, we have to take into account the obvious physiological barriers that affect Mr Smith's ability to communicate effectively, as well as receiving and analysing information in relation to his clinical status. The patient is also without an escort, who might have been able to provide more in-depth information, giving the nurse a fuller, more holistic picture. This in turn would promote and optimise the assessment and prioritisation of his nursing needs. It is clear Mr Smith is frightened and distressed and the issues are exacerbated by an angry and distressed relative. Many patients are scared when they seek care, and fear may colour their interactions (Pytel et al., 2009). This scenario poses a significant challenge for the nurse dealing with the situation. It is easy to become overwhelmed because of the vast array of information, so let's go back to basics!

We need to draw on our nursing experience and the fundamental underpinning philosophy of nursing, the nursing process. In the first instance, we need to undertake a nursing assessment of the situation, and highlight and prioritise the key points. While we are undertaking this assessment, we must ensure that we *talk* to the patient and *listen* to what information is being communicated back to us, by Mr Smith or his daughter. We will also have to *transmit* and *relay* information and may need to involve the multidisciplinary team members when implementing Mr Smith's care.

As with any interventions that are put in place, an evaluation of care must be undertaken and it is important that we do this effectively and safely. Therefore, a variety of media resources may be required. It is important that we communicate in a way that the patient understands. Previous studies have identified several nurse-related communication barriers: stereotyping, poor articulation and excessive use of medical terminology (Park and Song, 2005). Clinically, Mr Smith's neurological status is compromised and he needs nursing and medical interventions to be put in place to address his clinical needs, in this case hydration and pressure ulcer care, and management needs. Not only must we involve Mr Smith in his care, we must also involve his family and keep them informed as well, with the best information available. We might summarise the actions for Mr. Smith's management as below:

- reassure and orient the patient
- listen attentively to the relative and involve them in the patient's care
- enlist assistance of team members for medical assessment
- give simple explanation of events and interventions to the patient and relative together
- empower the relative to assist with rather than disrupt care-giving.

Dealing with conflict

Yoder-Wise (2019) suggests that:

> Conflict among health care providers is inevitable and is compounded by employee diversity, high nurse-to-patient ratios, pressure to make timely decisions and status differences.
>
> (Yoder-Wise, 2019:124)

There are many reasons why conflict may occur within an acute or critical care setting and some have been highlighted above. Bizek and Fontaine (2011) indicate that anxiety can be alleviated with simple explanations. In 2013, NHS Protect launched guidance on *Meeting Needs and Reducing Distress* (NHS Protect, 2013). The guidance discusses the consequences of not dealing with challenging behaviour effectively and discusses key points that include communication – talking and listening. The guidance emphasises the importance of positive engagement and communication when facing challenging behaviour.

As nurses working in acute care we must ensure that de-escalation techniques are adopted, not only to promote our own safety but also ensure that a peaceful outcome is met without any injuries being incurred. Indeed, conflict resolution training should factor into any professional and personal development plans discussed by your clinical leads to ensure that your communication skills remain current.

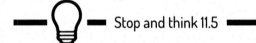 **Stop and think 11.5**

Can you identify two forms of communication that are likely to diffuse an aggressive situation or prevent such a situation? What rationale would you give for using these forms of communication in these situations? See Chapter 8 for possible answers.

Children and young people

Communicating with children or young people provides nurses in acute and critical care settings with a different set of challenges. You have to very quickly win over a child's trust, and build up a rapport and 'bond' with the child. Children may be very frightened, as clinical environments can look sterile, bright and inevitably noisy. Furthermore, dependent on their age, children may find it difficult to express themselves effectively. Equally, nurses need to take into account a child's previous experience of hospital that may not have been favourable.

In 2005, the Department for Education and Skills (DfES) worked collaboratively with a variety of service users, employers and worker interests to develop common core skills and knowledge for agencies who dealt with children and young people (DfES, 2005). The prospectus, updated in 2010, sets out the requirements for six areas of expertise, one of which was in relation to effective communication and engagement with children, young people, their families and carers (Children's Workforce Development Council, 2010).

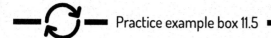 Practice example box 11.5

Communicating with a 2-year-old and their parent

Lucy is 2 years old. She has fallen, sustaining a cut to her arm, and is distressed on arrival. She is accompanied by her mother who is also upset as Lucy was in her care at the time of the accident.

Identify the communication skills required in this situation. How will you adapt or modify your communication skills to ensure that you maintain a high standard of care for Lucy and her mother? List the techniques you may use. Possible answers will be given in the text below.

A child who is in pain and distressed will be difficult to assess and manage. There are many techniques that professionals can engage in when assessing and managing pain in children. One example is the use of distraction techniques, with the inclusion of toys, music, books, games and play.

We need to take into account that Lucy *and* her mother are distressed. It will also be important to ascertain Lucy's understanding of the situation. Every care must be taken to ensure the correct information is elicited from Lucy and her mother. Additionally, there will be pressure to act quickly to alleviate Lucy's pain, although you must ensure any care that is given is done so in a safe and timely manner.

It is important to remember that children require a different set of skills, utilising appropriate family-friendly and indeed family-centred care models which encompass holistically the needs of the child and their families or significant others. Nurses should also be mindful of safeguarding the interests of the child.

Knowledge link See Chapter 13 for more on communicating with children and young people, and safeguarding their interests.

Patients with perceptual disturbance or confusion

Patients experiencing acute psychotic symptoms or disorientation are most likely to feel frightened by an unfamiliar environment and people they don't know. Such patients may lack understanding of what is happening around them or have a quite erroneous idea of where they are, who the staff members are and what people's intentions might be. People who are frightened and feel threatened are likely to become aggressive or withdrawn and unco-operative. Their understanding of verbal communication is often impaired because they may be distracted, have poor concentration or not be able to process whole sentences. A communication priority for these patients is to *help them feel safe*.

Earlier chapters have taken you through different communication methods and approaches so you should be able to apply these principles to practice and give a rationale for each approach. Look at the list in Table 11.1 and see if you can identify some key actions you could utilise with a patient with poor cognition and perceptual disturbance. Suggested actions are given in Table 11.2, below.

Table 11.1 Key actions by nurses for the patient with perceptual disturbance

Communication approach	To do	To avoid	Rationale
1 Body language			
2 Vocal style			
3 Verbal style			
4 Environment management			
5 Appearance			
6 Relationship building			

What patient behaviour would help you evaluate the effectiveness of your practice in this situation? There are lots of different approaches you may have identified but hopefully they will be those that aim to reduce distrust and improve the relationship between you and the patient.

Patients who cannot take in or respond to verbal reassurance and explanation will still be able to interpret the physical and human environment around them. When cognitive processing is impaired, people rely on emotional perception. If they feel fear, the environment will be interpreted as threatening. If helped to feel safe, the environment will be less scary. See Table 11.2 for some suggested actions.

Table 11.2 Key actions by nurses for the patient with perceptual disturbance

Communication approach	To do	To avoid	Rationale
1 Body language	Open posture Keep at eye level Keep your distance	Touching Quick movements Close proximity	Gives non-threatening and even submissive messages. Avoids increasing nervous arousal.
2 Vocal style	Quiet, reassuring tone, slow pace	Loudness, sudden or staccato speech	Patient will be aware you are speaking to them. They will hear your tone of voice.

3	Verbal style	Give information and commentary on what is happening. Keep it simple.	Not speaking, even if patient is unresponsive.	Reduce stressors. Aids relationship building.
4	Environment management	Remove threats (or remove *from* threats). Keep feared objects out of sight.	Interruptions, security staff, technical equipment, cameras, mobile phones and bleepers, sharps.	Electrical equipment is threatening to paranoid patients.
5	Appearance	Remove signs of authority. Smile. Wear a jumper or cardigan over uniform (more friendly).	Authoritarian or confusing clothes and accessories (keys, lapels, badges, male nurse tunics). Religious symbols (especially with acutely psychotic patients).	Reduces risk of being confused with controlling authorities. Patient needs to maintain a sense of control.
6	Relationship building	Active listening! Get person to talk, preferably, about themselves. Use familiar 'props', i.e. a cup of tea or hot chocolate, biscuits. Superficial self-disclosure.	Frequently leaving the patient. Too many people with the patient at any one time. Sending trusted relatives or friends away without good cause.	Psychotic and disoriented patients will 'invent' an explanation of their surroundings using human and environmental cues. Demonstrates empathy and human contact. All aim to develop trust.

Source: after Mason and Chandley, 1999; Duxbury, 2000

Knowledge link See Chapter 1 on the different theories of communication channels and Chapter 8 on de-escalation skills.

Communication skills for emergency situations

An emergency situation, such as a cardiac arrest, a fire or a patient being found injured, requires the nurse to act quickly and communicate effectively.

A patient's condition can change suddenly and the nurse's role is to ensure that any sudden changes are detected and communicated quickly so treatment can be implemented. The Acute Illness Management (AIM) programme (Greater Manchester Critical Care Skills Institute, 2015) equips nurses of all fields of care with the skills to recognise potentially life-threatening signs of deterioration in patients, hopefully preventing them from suffering a respiratory or cardiac arrest that may be fatal.

Part of the AIM programme focuses on communicating in an emergency and offers a framework – situation, background, assessment and recommendation (or SBAR) – for ensuring that the information relayed is effective and produces the required response from whoever it is being communicated to. The SBAR tool originated in the US Navy and was later adapted for use in healthcare. This framework is utilised across the NHS for reporting incidents and emergency situations (NHS Institute for Innovation and Improvement, 2010).

It provides a systematic approach to reporting information in an emergency and ensuring that the facts are communicated appropriately and effectively, preventing a delay in treatment for the patient or an inappropriate response to the emergency.

Table 11.3   The principles of SBAR to be used when reporting an incident or emergency

Situation	• Who you are • Exact location • The patient's name • State the problem or identify the nature of the incident
Background	Give brief details relating to the patient's history, i.e. date/time of admission, diagnosis, summary of treatment and any other relevant medical history.
Assessment	State your assessment of the patient using the ABCDE* approach and include current vital signs, mental state, fluid balance, and track and trigger score. Provide relevant and specific data which identifies the exact condition of the patient.
Recommendation	• Explain what you need from the person you are reporting to. • Be specific about your request and the timeframe. • Ask if there is anything else you can do before the other person arrives. • Document the call including date, time and who you spoke to.

*See Table 11.6 for an explanation of the ABCDE approach.

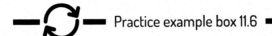 Practice example box 11.6

Mrs James

Mrs James, aged 45, has been admitted to the medical assessment unit with pneumonia. On admission she was dyspnoeic with a respiratory rate of 36 breaths/min and pyrexial temperature 38.5°C. You are asked by the staff nurse to complete some observations on her but when you go to her bed you find Mrs James to be restless and agitated. Her blood pressure is 90/60 mmHg and her pulse is 110 beats/min, with a respiratory rate is 40 breaths/min. She is responsive to voice but is clearly confused.

As a student nurse you call for help and the staff nurse asks you to go and phone the doctor.

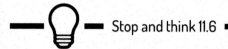

Stop and think 11.6

Look at Practice example box 11.6. Using the SBAR framework, identify the information you will need to give to the doctor when you call them to ensure an effective response and that the best interests of the patient are met. Table 11.4 gives a suggested answer.

Table 11.4 Suggested answer for Stop and think 11.6

Situation	• Who you are • Medical assessment unit • Patient: Mrs James • Patient is confused
Background	Admitted with pneumonia, dyspnoeic on admission, no prior medical history and wasn't confused on admission.
Assessment	She is breathing; her respiratory rate has increased from 36 to 40 breaths/min. Her blood pressure is 90/60 mmHg and her pulse is 110 beats/min. Her temperature is 38.5°C and she responds to voice but is confused.
Recommendation	• You will ask the doctor to attend urgently to assess the patient. • You will ask if there is anything the doctor wishes you to do for the patient while you are waiting for them to arrive. • Document date, time and who you spoke to in the nursing notes.

Team communication in an emergency

When an emergency occurs (such as when resuscitating a patient, as in Table 11.4), someone needs to take charge of the situation and direct the other people involved in the incident. There are no general rules about who that person should be as long as they manage the situation effectively and work within their scope of practice (NMC, 2018). Even junior nurses may have to take control of an emergency situation and manage it until someone more senior or more qualified arrives to help.

Teams are only effective if they have an effective leader and, in an emergency, it is paramount that the person who takes control is calm and in control of the situation. This will ensure that the other staff involved feel confident and assured. For example, effective resuscitations occur when all those involved know exactly what their role is and what is expected of them.

Adair (1979), cited by Mullins (2011), identifies three areas of need within a working team and suggests that the effectiveness of a team is entirely dependent on how effective the leader is at meeting these three areas of need (Table 11.5).

Table 11.5 Adair's three areas of need outline effective team working in an emergency situation

1 Task function

- Achieving the specific objectives of resuscitating the patient.
- Planning the resuscitation and allocating roles within the team.
- Controlling the resuscitation and monitoring performance of the team members ensuring a systematic approach is followed (ABCDE*).
- Reviewing progress at various points through the systematic process.

2 Team function

- Maintaining morale throughout and reassuring the team members.
- Ensuring standards are maintained (UK resuscitation guidelines adhered to).
- Providing effective communication throughout the resuscitation and directing individuals to perform specific roles at appropriate times.
- Ensuring that each member of the team is respected and valued.

3 Individual functions

- Providing feedback and debrief opportunity at the end of the resuscitation for the staff involved.
- Ensuring any staff training or individual needs are identified and managed appropriately.
- Providing information and support to the family of the patient.
- Reconciling any conflict which may have arisen within the team if the resuscitation was problematic or unsuccessful in outcome.

*See Table 11.6 for an explanation of the ABCDE approach.

Source: Adair, 1979 cited by Mullins, 2011

In terms of working as a team in assessing and managing a critically ill or injured patient, the most effective team works simultaneously in a process known as **horizontal organisation** (Driscoll et al., 2003). For tasks to be performed simultaneously there needs to be effective allocation of roles and responsibilities as identified in Table 11.5. Each person within the team must understand what tasks need to be performed and in what sequence, and the role of the team leader is to oversee that the process occurs according to the specific protocol being used.

Using the example of a patient who has been involved in a road traffic collision and is unconscious on admission, the team will complete a systematic assessment of the patient using the ABCDE approach (see Table 11.6). The ABCDE approach, which stands for airway and cervical spine control, breathing, circulation, disability/deformity and exposure, is a systematic approach for immediate assessment to provide life-saving aid.

Table 11.6 ABCDE: a systematic approach to patient assessment

A	Airway and cervical spine control
B	Breathing
C	Circulation
D	Disability/deformity
E	Exposure

Nurses within the team will be assigned various roles associated with a specific part of the systematic assessment. The team leader will co-ordinate the assessment and collate all the information received from the team relating to the status of the patient; i.e. is the airway secure? What are their vital signs and their neurological status? Information will be gathered and communicated to other members of the healthcare team to instigate treatment, make referrals or order investigations. The most important aspect of this kind of teamwork is that all those involved will be communicating continuously while monitoring the patient or delivering care or treatment. The team will work together to achieve a common goal, which is essentially to do their best for the patient.

Situations such as these can be extremely stressful for all involved, including the relatives of the patient. Effective communication is required between the team leader and the nurse who is caring for the relatives so that they can be kept informed and involved in the decision-making process. Relatives are often encouraged where appropriate to remain with their loved one while the resuscitation is carried out. This can be stressful for them and the team but can be beneficial for the relatives if supported appropriately throughout by the team.

If we look back at the practice example of Mr Smith in Practice example box 11.4., we can see that involving the relative in the patient's care empowers the relative and distracts her from expressing her anger and interrupting the care team.

The resuscitation of children will almost always involve parents being with their child and this can be a very emotional experience for all involved. It is vital in these situations that the nurse remains with the relatives and is not involved in the actual resuscitation. Relatives may be traumatised by the situation they observe and may have lots of questions, or none at all, and the nurse must be sensitive to their needs and their anxieties.

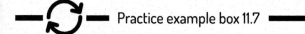 Practice example box 11.7

Mr Robertson

A 60-year-old man comes into the emergency department following a cardiac arrest at home. His 24-year-old son James, who has learning disabilities, accompanies him and is extremely distressed. He wants to stay with his father and so a nurse takes him into the resuscitation room and stays with him while the resuscitation team carry out the resuscitation.

Consider the effect that James being present in the room may have on the resuscitation team. How can the nurse support James throughout this process and what factors may need to be considered in relation to communication with him?

Suggested answer: the nurse can support James by ensuring they give a full explanation of the resuscitation and what is happening to his father using simple terms and ensuring James

(Continued)

understands (answering questions fully). The nurse should pre-empt the sequence of resuscitation so they can prepare James for any invasive procedures. They should attempt to get someone who he knows to come to be with him to provide support, and ensure he knows he can leave the room if he wants. They can also offer refreshments but stay with him at all times. The nurse should allow James to hold his father's hand when appropriate. The team need to acknowledge that they are engaging in a witnessed resuscitation and that James may have difficulties comprehending questions or events.

There are a number of issues to be considered in relation to communicating in an emergency situation either as an individual nurse or as a member of a team. The nurse must be able to respond quickly and identify the priorities for information giving and ensure that the information relayed is acted upon to safeguard the interests of the patient.

Conclusion

This chapter has considered some of the complex and challenging issues that student nurses will inevitably face in acute and critical care. Many of the issues require nurses to think, act and communicate quickly with a wide variety of patients and professionals. Very often it will be the nurse who is the starting point for any communication process that is required. As such, selection and justification of appropriate communication approaches are essential to promote patient safety and, where possible, facilitate a positive experience for the family and significant others.

FURTHER READING

Conflict Resolution. www.instituteofconflictmanagement.org/.
Critical Care Skills Institute. http://gmccn.org.uk/education.
Resuscitation Council. www.resus.org.uk/siteindx.htm.
Royal College of Nursing Emergency Care Association. www.rcn.org.uk/get-involved/
   forums/emergency-care-association.
Royal College of Paediatrics and Child Health. www.rcpch.ac.uk/.

REFERENCES

Alvarez, G. and Coiera, E. (2005) Interruptive communication patterns in the intensive care unit ward round. *International Journal of Medical Informatics*, 74, 791–796.
Bizek, K.S. and Fontaine, D.K. (2011) The patient's experience with critical illness. In P.G. Morton and D.K. Fontaine (eds), *Critical Care Nursing: A Holistic Approach* (11th edn). Philadelphia, Lippincott, Williams & Wilkins.

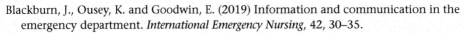

Blackburn, J., Ousey, K. and Goodwin, E. (2019) Information and communication in the emergency department. *International Emergency Nursing*, 42, 30–35.

Brown, A.F.T. and Cadogan, M.D. (2016) *Emergency Medicine: Diagnosis and Management* (7th edn). London, CRC Press.

Children's Workforce Development Council (2010) *The Common Core of Skills and Knowledge: At the Heart of What You Do.* Leeds, Children's Workforce Development Council.

DfES (2005) *Common Core of Skills and Knowledge for the Children's Workforce: Every Child Matters: Change for Children.* Nottingham, DfES Publications.

Dolan, B. and Holt. L. (2013) *Accident & Emergency: Theory into Practice* (3rd edn). London, Balliere Tindall Elsevier.

Driscoll, P.A., Gwinnutt, C.L., LeDuc Jimmerson, C. and Goodall, O. (2003) *Trauma Resuscitation: The Team Approach* (2nd edn). London, Bios Scientific Publishers.

Duxbury, J. (2000) *Difficult Patients.* Oxford, Butterworth-Heinemann.

Greater Manchester Critical Care Skills Institute (2015) *Acute Illness Management (AIM) Course Manual* (5th edn). Manchester, AIM.

Manchester Triage Group (2013) *Emergency Triage* (3rd edn). Oxford, John Wiley & Sons.

Mason, T. and Chandley, M. (1999) *Managing Violence and Aggression: A Manual for Nurses and Health Care Workers.* Edinburgh, Churchill Livingstone.

Mullins, L.J. (2011) *Management and Organisational Behaviour* (11th edn). New York, Pearson Education.

NHS Institute for Innovation and Improvement (2010) *Safer Care SBAR: Implementation and Training Guide.* Coventry, NHS Institute for Innovation and Improvement.

NHS Protect (2013) *Meeting Needs and Reducing Distress: Guidance on the Prevention and Management of Clinically Related Challenging Behaviour in NHS Settings.* London, NHS Protect.

NMC (2018) *The Code: Professional Standards of Practice and Behaviour for Nurses, Midwives and Nursing Associates.* www.nmc.org.uk/standards/code/.

Park, E.K. and Song, M. (2005) Communication barriers perceived by older patients and nurses. *International Journal of Nursing Studies*, 42, 59–166.

Parkinson, K., Newbury-Birch, D., Phillipson, A., Hindmarch, P., Kaner, E., Stamp, E., Vale, L., Wright, J. and Connolly, J. (2016) Prevalence of alcohol related attendance at an inner city emergency department and its impact: a dual prospective and retrospective cohort study. *Emergency Medicine Journal*, 33, 187–193.

Pierre, M., Hofinger, G. and Buerschaper, C. (2007) *Crisis Management in Acute Care Settings: Human Factors and Team Psychology in a High Stakes Environment.* London, Springer.

Pytel, C., Fielden, N.M., Meyer, K.H. and Albert, N. (2009) Nurse-patient/visitor communication in the emergency department. *Journal of Emergency Nursing*, 35(5), 406–411.

Yoder-Wise, P.S. (2019) *Leading and Managing in Nursing* (7th edn). St Louis, MO, Mosby.

TWELVE
COMMUNICATING WITH PEOPLE WITH CHRONIC AND LONG-TERM HEALTH NEEDS

GARY WITHAM

THIS CHAPTER WILL HELP YOU TO ACHIEVE
....COMPETENCIES IN:

- Being proactive and creative in enhancing communication and understanding
- Using appropriate communication skills to deal with difficult and challenging circumstances
- Promoting health and wellbeing, self-care and independence
- Discussing sensitive issues in relation to public health and death and dying

Introduction

A positive aspect to improving healthcare is that, across the world, people are living longer (WHO, 2018). Unfortunately, this does not always mean living a healthy older age. In England, those living with long-term conditions are intensive users of the NHS, using 50% of all GP appointments, 64% of all outpatient appointments and over 70% of all inpatient bed days (Department of Health, 2012). It is forecast that by 2035 there will be a 148% increase in people over 85 in England, and a large number of those people will have complex care needs (Kingston et al., 2018). While the older population is increasingly healthy, many are living with chronic illnesses such as diabetes, cardiovascular disease, arthritis, depression, dementia and co-morbidities (Goodwin et al., 2010; PHE, 2018).

Patients living with chronic illness learn to adapt and manage themselves in ways that meet their day-to-day needs. Their contact with healthcare professionals is often brief and so it is in this context that nurses may engage with this diverse patient group, as the following quote reinforces:

> Even people with long term conditions, who tend to be heavy users of the health service, are likely to spend less than 1% of their time in contact with health professionals. The rest of the time they, their carers and their families manage on their own.
>
> (Department of Health, 2014:12)

Self-care and self-management are therefore an integral part of UK government health policy (Department of Health, 2014). In supporting patients and facilitating this patient-centred approach, effective communication becomes a key component in patient care. The requirement to provide targeted information (Department of Health, 2006) appropriate to an individual's needs necessitates the establishment of professional relationships based on effective communication. The End of Life Care Strategy (Department of Health, 2008) suggests bereavement information and support should be available as part of end-of-life care provision and, in particular, recommends communication as an essential element of workforce training (Department of Health, 2008:118). The National Service Framework for long-term conditions (Department of Health, 2005) and other guidance (Department of Health, 2010) also highlight effective communication as an essential workforce requirement in supporting patients and carers.

In this chapter we will explore the different ways to relate to people living with chronic illness. We will examine issues of self-care and behavioural change, eliciting patient concerns, handling bad or significant news and dealing with loss and bereavement. In the context of chronic disease, exchanging information, managing uncertainty and the adoption of health-promoting behaviours are important issues.

Identifying patient concerns

Facilitating good self-care requires a relationship of trust that will sustain long-term clinical relationships and the provision of individualised health information and advice. The patient is the expert; therefore, nurses need to be sensitive in providing support and advice about flexible and realistic interventions for people living with chronic disease. Identifying patient concerns, especially with many patients managing complex needs, is a vital component of nurse assessment.

However, valuing patient experience can be difficult during a clinical consultation. Giving time to listen and identify the patient's main concerns allows the patient to share their experiences.

Look at the example in Box 12.1 of an exchange between a nurse and patient, who is living with chronic obstructive pulmonary disease (COPD), during an assessment:

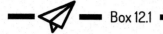 Box 12.1

Nurse/patient dialogue 1

Nurse: 'Hi Betty, have you been sleeping OK and are your bowels working?'

Betty: 'Err, they're OK thank you.'

Nurse: 'You seem upset. Is there anything wrong?'

Betty: 'I've been thinking about the future. I've been coping well but things are getting worse and I'm worried about what this all means.'

Nurse: 'Don't worry; it's understandable that you're concerned. I think a lot of people in your shoes feel this way. Often the worry goes once the treatment starts and you begin to feel better. I can get a doctor to give you information about the treatment if that would help.'

Betty: 'I don't really want to bother the doctor, err, don't worry. I'll be alright.'

Nurse: 'I know it must be difficult, what does your husband feel about the situation?'

Betty: 'Well he's obviously concerned, I think it's difficult for all of us. I'm worried but I've always been the strong one and I don't want to alarm the family.'

Nurse: 'Oh I see, do you have a big family?'

Betty: 'Yes, I have three daughters, and four granddaughters. They're very good and live close to me.'

Nurse: 'That's nice, to have that support around you, I suspect that's a great help isn't it? I've just got to go and do something else but can I quickly ask you if your appetite is OK?'

Betty: 'Yes.'

Nurse: 'Thanks, that's all the questions on my assessment form. I'll catch up with you later.'

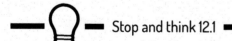 Stop and think 12.1

Can you identify verbal behaviours and actions by the nurse in the dialogue in Box 12.1 that prevent Betty from sharing her concerns?

From the interview you may have identified the following examples of behaviours that block open communication:

a   Closed questions ('Can I ask if your appetite is OK?')
b   Multiple questions ('Have you been sleeping OK and are your bowels working?')
c   Switching the person ('How does your husband feel about that?')
d   Leading questions ('I suspect that's a great help isn't it?')
e   Passing the buck ('I can get a doctor to give you information.')
f   Minimising or normalising comments ('I think a lot of people in your shoes feel that way.')
g   Premature reassurance ('Don't worry.')
h   Premature or inappropriate advice ('Often the worry goes once the treatment starts and you begin to feel better.')
i   Overt blocking ('Oh, I see, do you have a big family?').

The next dialogue (Box 12.2) involves the same assessment but the responses are handled differently.

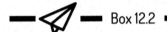 Box 12.2

Nurse/patient dialogue 2

Nurse: 'Hi Betty, how are you feeling?'

Betty: 'Err, well, I'm OK really.'

Nurse: 'You seem upset. Is there anything wrong?'

Betty: 'I've been thinking about the future. I've been coping well but things are getting worse and I'm worried about what this all means.'

Nurse: 'What are you worried about?'

Betty: 'I've coped well with my lung problems but getting more out of puff and I can't really do things I could do 6 months ago. Shopping's getting difficult. The doctor did say that there was not too much that could be done about it.'

Nurse: 'What did you understand by what she said?'

Betty: 'Well it's obviously concerning. I don't know how long things are going to continue. I know I can't go on like this. I think it's difficult for all of us. I'm worried but I've always been the strong one and I don't want to alarm the family.'

Nurse: 'That sounds really difficult.' (silence)

Betty: 'Yes.' (visibly upset)

Nurse: 'Is it difficult being the strong one?'

Betty: 'Yes, I just can't do the cooking, shopping or at times walk up the stairs. I don't think I can cope.'

Nurse: 'What does "not coping" mean to you?'

Betty: 'I'll have to just let things go. I find it very difficult.'

Nurse: 'I can see. Can you bear to tell me any other thoughts that you have had?'

Betty: 'I think how to talk to my husband about it all, he doesn't like to dwell on things.'

Nurse: 'So, can I check that I've understood, you are worried about what the future holds because your breathing is worse. This is affecting how you're coping at home with the shopping, cooking and getting around and you're worried how to talk to your husband?'

Betty: 'Yes.'

Nurse: 'Anything else worrying you?'

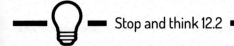 Stop and think 12.2

Can you identify verbal behaviours and actions that allowed Betty to share her concerns? From the interview you may have identified the following examples of behaviours that encourage and facilitate open communication:

a   Open questions ('How are you feeling?')
b   Empathy ('That sounds really difficult.')
c   Open directive questions ('What did you understand by what she said?')
d   Negotiation ('Can you bear to tell me any other thoughts?')
e   Questions with a psychological focus ('Is it difficult being the strong one?')
f   Questions with cognitive focus ('Tell me any other thoughts.')
g   Checking understanding and summarising ('So, can I check that I've understood, you are worried ...')
h   Clarifying psychological cues ('What does "not coping" mean to you?')
i   Screening questions to explore other concerns ('Anything else worrying you?').

Nurses need to be sensitive to patient cues that arise during communication. Patient cues can be defined as:

Words or phrases suggesting vague undefined emotions, verbal hints to hidden concerns, mention of psychological symptoms, neutral mention of an important life event and repetition of a previous neutral expression. Non-verbal cues include expression of emotion: crying or hints of emotion: sighing, frowning.

(Del Piccolo et al., 2006)

Patients are much more likely to tell nurses of their concerns if the nurse asks questions with a psychological focus in the presence of a cue. In our scenario, for example, the nurse notices Betty is upset and asks if there is anything wrong. The important element is to respond to that initial cue. A patient who needs to share a significant concern will often target a particular student or staff nurse rather than asking the first person who comes along. Therefore, taking the question/cue seriously will often develop the trust necessary to explore the concern (Gorawara-Bhat et al., 2017). There is evidence that picking up cues actually shortens consultation time (Butow et al., 2002) and reduces anxiety (Zwingmann et al., 2017).

In clarifying the patient's concerns, it is important to maintain a psychological focus since evidence suggests that nurses' communication tends to be related to physical issues rather than an exploration of the patient's feelings (Kruijver et al., 2001). Many nurses may feel it is difficult to explore patient concerns for a number of reasons.

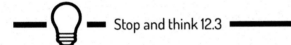 Stop and think 12.3

Can you think of the reasons why health professionals find exploring patient concerns difficult?

Some evidence suggests that, as nurses, we may fear that exploring issues with patients would take up too much time, that we may be faced with answering emotionally difficult questions, or that we might get 'out of our depth' (Friedrichsen and Milberg, 2006; Delgado et al., 2017). Sometimes our beliefs play a role, for example, that emotional problems are just a 'natural' reaction to advancing disease, or that just talking is not going to fix anything and it's not really our role to explore these concerns. There may be issues of privacy on a busy ward or in someone's home with friends or family present. We may feel we lack training or peer support and therefore actively avoid more meaningful interactions. We may also be afraid of over-stepping the 'boundaries' of professional behaviour and getting 'too involved'.

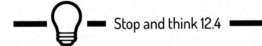 Stop and think 12.4

Can you think of the reasons why patients may not talk about their concerns?

Some patients may feel they would be a burden to the nurse and do not want to upset them. Others may feel that nurses are too busy and that other patients' needs are greater than their own concerns. Patients may also be sensitive to the environment in which they are in; fear of getting upset on a busy ward with limited privacy may limit the disclosure of concerns. There may also be cultural and language barriers or nurses may block patient cues and focus only on medical aspects of care. This again may prevent disclosure. This is an important issue since most NHS environments are focused on medical treatment rather than psychosocial support. The physical focus of the medical model of care, often associated with attempts at curing the ill patient, can make talk about 'feelings' very difficult for patients. People living with chronic disease, including mental illness and learning difficulty, may not fit into a system where cure and medical treatment are not always appropriate. However, they may still have important concerns that are not being addressed by health professionals.

Breaking bad or significant news

Breaking bad or significant news can be difficult. The reasons can be similar to talking about patient concerns: the fear of upsetting a patient, not being able to 'handle' the situation or causing the patient harm. There is also the need for acceptance that as a nurse there are some situations where we cannot make things 'better' and need to sit physically and sometimes emotionally with the patient through the conveying of difficult news. It is often the case that a doctor will break bad news, especially if it centres on treatment decisions, but it is also important to remember that it may be difficult for a patient to take in all the implications or information at once. Therefore, you may be the person a patient will ask to 'unpack' the meaning of the information they have been given.

Sometimes doctors adopt a number of strategies to avoid the impact of breaking bad news. These strategies include lengthy information-giving or explanation, using complicated words, recommending another type of treatment, referring the patient to another department or suggesting discontinued treatment (Shaw et al., 2015). These avoidance strategies make it difficult for patients to understand the implications of what is being said and lead to the patient feeling dissatisfied with the breaking of bad news by doctors (Spiegel et al., 2009). Current practice in breaking significant news often increases the patient's unmet concerns and leads to increased anxiety (see Figure 12.1 for an illustration of this). In the longer term this can lead to higher emotional distress associated with anxiety and depressive illness.

We will examine the SPIKES model for breaking significant news. The important element is checking the patient's anticipation of the information you will give them. Does the patient actually want the information and, if expects, warn them about it first. It is better to give information in small chunks and in you are unsure what the patient language that a patient will understand. After giving the information, look for cues in their emotional response. How does the patient feel about what was said? What is their understanding?

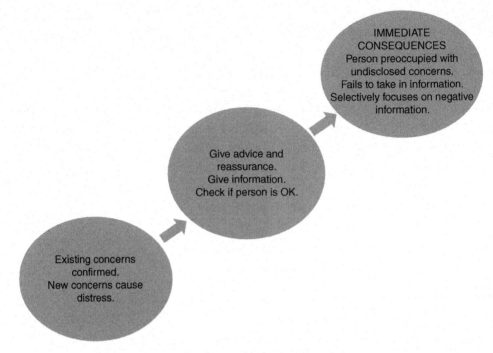

Figure 12.1 An example of current practice in breaking significant news

This part is important in responding to the emotional impact and patient concerns with the breaking of significant news. Towards the end of the discussion it can be helpful to summarise the main points and clarify that this understanding is shared by the patient. At this stage a plan can be negotiated with the patient to address their concerns and expectations and offer the appropriate support. It is important to offer written information to back up the verbal information given and to include relevant contact numbers.

The SPIKES Model

Communication guidelines for breaking bad news in the United States are incorporated in the Education for Physicians on End-of-Life Care (EPEC). This is a six-step approach based on the SPIKES model, which stands for setting, perception, invitation, knowledge, empathy and strategy/summary (Wittenberg-Lyles et al., 2008):

1 prepare for the interaction (setting)
2 assess knowledge base (perception; ask-before-you-tell principle)
3 gauge/negotiate the amount of information the patient wants (invitation)
4 deliver bad news (knowledge)
5 physician response to bad news (empathy)
6 summary involving discussing the follow-up plan.

The setting is an important component of sharing bad news, and in working with medical colleagues it may be left to the nurse to identify the appropriate area to talk to patients and/or relatives. It can often be the first non-verbal trigger that significant information is to be shared and therefore can be a warning sign to patients/relatives that important information is to be exchanged. After the initial medical consultation is over the patient/relative may have many questions. These can occur over a longer time frame and you as the nurse may be the first point of contact for the patient. Remember to reflect back to the patient to ascertain their understanding of the information, for example:

'What do you understand by what Dr Smith told you?'

'What do you know about your current situation?'

Never assume that the patient knows their prognosis, or is aware of new significant information about their condition (even if nursing/medical notes indicate a discussion has taken place). The patient may not have processed certain information and breaking significant news can be better viewed as a process rather than a focus on one central piece of information or consultation. Sometimes it involves communication 'clean up' with patients who have not shared honest diagnosis/prognosis talk with previous doctors (Wittenberg-Lyles et al., 2008).

Patients or relatives may ask the same questions to different health professionals. It is important for trust and consistency to be honest and open about the level of information you can give. If you are unsure of the answers, say so and, if appropriate, ask the person why they are asking that particular question. This can help you understand the reasons why patients/relatives may be checking the consistency of the information given and allow you to further 'unpack' the issues and offer support.

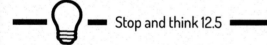 Stop and think 12.5

What are the reasons why patients sometimes do not acknowledge the reality of significant events or situations?

Denial

Denial can be associated with improved psychological functioning and can be helpful if the denial is an active strategy. For example, one might realise that one has cancer but choose not to let that diagnosis control one's life by ignoring the illness and creating a positive outlook. Denial can also relate to poorer psychological functioning by the adoption of passive strategies, for example refusing to believe it has happened or hoping for a miracle (Vos and de Haes, 2007). A patient who has been given significant news, such as a poor prognosis, may not be ready to process that information. It may be too difficult to explore or imagine. The function of denial is to protect the patient against intolerable distress. Denial of the reality of death can generate difficulties for the patient or relative to work through important emotional and practical aspects of living with a life-limiting condition. The subsequent 'unfinished business' can lead to a more complicated bereavement process. When supporting a patient in complete denial, it is important to acknowledge the protective nature of this mechanism and that direct confrontation may not be the best approach. It is a powerful psychological defence unlikely to be broken by sensitive probing or exploration.

If the denial is not complete then it may be appropriate for the health professional to reassess their denial status; to explore this area to open up discussion. In order to gauge the level of denial, one can try challenging any inconsistencies in the patient's or relative's story:

'You told me that the surgery wasn't significant. But how do you feel about the fact that you have been recovering for 3 months and may need more treatment?'

A nurse can also check if the denial is total by seeing if there is a 'window' on the denial:

'I wonder if there was a time you felt that things were not going to be OK?'

'Can you possibly share those feelings?'

'Can you bear to go any further?'

Collusion

The relative

Relatives will sometimes try to protect themselves and the patient from the impending loss related to end-stage illness. This can involve not disclosing information about the prognosis to a patient and requesting that health professionals collude in this by withholding the truth. This can affect the trust between nurse and patient and lead to communication difficulties. Certain subject areas can become 'off limits', restricting the dialogue of important issues at the end of life. In dealing with collusion the first step is to talk with the relative responsible for the collusion. How are they coping with the present situation? Is it taking an emotional toll? If they give you any cues, try to establish the extent of the strain. Avoid minimising the situation or answering your own questions since the person may feel torn between an awareness of the impact of the disease and a strong wish to avoid facing it and maintaining the pretence. The nurse could then check if the collusion is affecting the relative's relationship with the patient. This may establish if it is affecting the communication between them and the subsequent impact on the colluder.

It is important to identify why the relative feels collusion is in their relative's interest and gauge the strength of those beliefs (without judging their rationale). The nurse can summarise the cost to the colluder and ask permission to check the patient's awareness of the present situation. Establish the 'ground rules' with the relative noting that, if the patient has no insight into their current situation, you will not give them new information.

The patient

The second step would be to talk to the patient and check their understanding of the situation. How do they interpret what is happening to them and how do they feel about it? You may find that the patient often has more awareness than the relative thinks they do and this gentle probing can sometimes lead to more open communication. Where both parties are trying to protect each other from distress, this intervention can subsequently allow them to explore their feelings.

If you can then negotiate an open discussion with the relative and patient as a third step then you can recap on what has been discussed, acknowledge the distress and check if they wish to talk, either alone or with you present. More open communication can be encouraged by the relative and patient, identifying each concern and working through it with dialogue.

Dealing with loss and bereavement

Loss and bereavement are difficult for nurses to communicate since we cannot make things 'better'. We may need to navigate through the intense personal experience of loss in a cathartic approach.

....

Knowledge link See Chapter 3 for Heron's six-category intervention analysis on cathartic interventions.

....

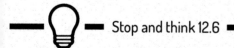 **Stop and think 12.6**

Think of a time in your clinical practice in which a patient was dying or had died.

- How did it make you feel?
- Did you find it easy to speak with family and friends about the death?
- How did you or other staff communicate with the friends and family of the patient who died?

In Box 12.3 Joan Didion describes her personal experience of grief at the sudden loss of her husband. It highlights the isolation and intensity of loss experienced by the bereaved and the attempt to make sense of loss in the narrative of their lives. A question many recently bereaved people ask is 'am I going mad?' Talking of the normality of such reactions as Didion's can be very supportive to the bereaved.

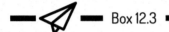 **Box 12.3**

Example of the experience of bereavement

Grief turns out to be a place none of us know until we reach it. We know that someone close to us could die. We might expect to feel shock. We do not expect this shock to be obliterative, dislocating to both body and mind. We might expect to be prostrate, inconsolable, crazy with loss. We do not expect to be literally crazy, cool customers who believe that their husband is about to return and need his shoes. Nor can we know ahead of the fact – and here lies the heart of the difference between grief as we imagine it and grief as it is – the unending absence that follows, the void, the relentless succession of moments during which we will confront the experience of meaninglessness itself.

(Didion, 2005:188)

There are many theoretical models of the grieving process, such as Bowlby and Parkes (1970), who identify four main stages in the grief process, Kubler-Ross (1970) in her seminal work *On Death and Dying*, in which she identifies five stages, and Worden (1991), who examines four 'tasks' of mourning.

....

Knowledge link See the reference list in this chapter for further reading and source books on these models of the grieving process.

....

Walter (1996) challenges these grand narratives. He describes the journey of the bereaved as one of trying to construct a narrative that incorporates the dead person within the structure of their lives, and that will continue to endure through time. The construction of a biography is vital to the incorporation of the memory of the dead into the bereaved person's continuing life. This process is developed, according to Walter, by conversation with others who knew the deceased. There is no 'closure' and 'resolution of grief'. Therefore, it is important for health professionals to give the grieving person the opportunity to talk about their loved one and describe the meaning and impact that the deceased had in their lives. This is a difficult process, as Mallon (2008) comments:

> There are no easy formulas for dealing with grief and bereavement. Each person has to live with it, live through it and grow through it. There are no fixed person times for its duration, despite theories of time-bound grief models, nor are there certainties about when or if understanding or acceptance will occur. Responding with sensitivity and care and holding the emotions of the bereaved as they travel through their grief are essentially healing aspects of our work.
>
> (Mallon, 2008:15)

There may be other factors that affect grief and the grieving process. The person's previous experience of death, the nature of the relationship (attachment), the circumstances of the death and the social support network will all have an impact. In terms of our role as a nurse, it can be difficult to sit with the pain of grief from the patient's significant others as well as dealing with our own feelings and emotions. If we have built up a relationship with the patient it can be hard not to be overwhelmed by the stressful event. It is important to remember that just your presence can be valued since it provides someone who will listen, who has known the patient and family and can acknowledge their grief. If there is ongoing contact with relatives it can put any feelings of guilt they may have into words, for example, 'could I have done anything differently?', and provides consolation in their loneliness (Holdsworth, 2015). In terms of your own feelings and emotions it is important to acknowledge them and it can be helpful to share those feelings with colleagues in the clinical environment you work in. By 'unpacking' the situation it can be a way to acknowledge the tragic, stressful event and give you the opportunity to talk about anything in particular that was significant for you.

Ambiguous loss: dementia

Loss and bereavement can also be seen in terms of accepting the changes that occur when living with chronic and long-term conditions. The changes in family roles in the presence of chronic illness can disrupt social functioning. One example is a family member living with dementia. The term 'ambiguous loss' (Boss, 1999) can often be described in this situation where there exists unfinished business in which the family of a person living with dementia have to adjust to 'losing' their family member (in terms of cognitive/psychological functioning) before death. Health professionals need to offer time, and engage with people encountering the continuing loss of a loved one.

In communicating with someone living with dementia it is important to acknowledge the importance of body language and non-verbal cues. Language may be affected as the person becomes increasingly unable to interpret the world in a way that makes sense to them. This can lead to misunderstandings and communication difficulties that can be frustrating for both the person living with dementia and those around them. Therefore tense, agitated facial expressions or movements may upset the person trying to understand what you want to communicate. Remaining calm, giving your full attention and remaining below their eye level rather than standing above them may create a safe environment where feelings may be expressed, even in the absence of language. When speaking, use simple, short sentences, allowing time for the person to process what has been said. Try not to ask the person to make complicated decisions that could cause confusion or frustration. If the person's conversation is not based in reality, try to respond in a way that does not cut off dialogue, or be too grounded in reality. For example, if a person states that she needs to go home to look after the baby, acknowledge that once she was a mother with a small baby and ask her about that time in her life.

Self-care and behavioural change

Cognitive behavioural therapy

We now look at a common approach to managing chronic disease: cognitive behavioural therapy (CBT). CBT examines the cause and effect within ourselves related to the decisions we make. Specific behaviours can relate to four interactive elements: physical sensation, behaviour, thoughts and emotions. How these elements interplay can affect a person's way of dealing with a situation. For example, Tim has chronic back pain but wants to go swimming. On this day, his back pain is particularly bad and he is unable to get out of the house. Tim may think his day has been spoiled, so his emotional reaction will be negative. Physically, he may experience loss of energy and increased pain and his behaviour may become restless and aimless. Alternatively, if Tim can plan a more achievable activity, then the emotional reaction of being unable to swim can be modified by thoughts about achieving another goal, so produce a physical response of improved energy leading to behavioural changes to achieve the new goal. Tim's response is generated by the meaning he attaches to the circumstances he finds himself in.

The style of communication in CBT often involves note-taking in an interview setting. Educating the patient in the cognitive behavioural approach is important, and engaging the patient in self-care is an important patient-centred aspect of CBT. Goal-/contract-setting provides a framework in CBT, highlighting the methods to be used by the therapist and the commitment by the patient in applying them. The sessions often remain structured and involve agenda review, homework feedback, a discussion of the next topic from treatment plan and homework setting.

In terms of the evidence base and chronic illness, CBT can be effective in improving quality of life of patients living with cancer (Duncan et al., 2017) and breast cancer in particular (Ye et al., 2018). It can be effective in cardiac rehabilitation to reduce anxiety and depression (Tully et al., 2015) as well as supporting people with multiple sclerosis and depression (Hind et al., 2014). It can also offer an improved outcome for people with chronic pain (Ostelo et al., 2005).

Knowledge link See Chapter 7 for further explanation of CBT and explanation of negative thinking patterns.

Motivational interviewing

Motivational interviewing (MI) can be defined as 'a client-centred, directive method for enhancing intrinsic motivation to change by exploring and resolving ambivalence' (Miller and Rollnick, 2002). The essential elements of MI are to attempt to change patient ambivalence, which can be a barrier to health behaviour change.

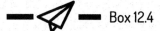 **Box 12.4**

Example of a clinic review

Peter is 50 years old and lives with his wife. He has a busy life working long, stressful hours for an insurance company. He is overweight and has a poor diet. A life-long smoker (20 a day), Peter was diagnosed with COPD 2 years ago after persistent breathing difficulties. He attends clinic for a review every 6 months but feels he is getting more breathless.

Box 12.4 outlines a typical case scenario of chronic illness associated with behaviour. There are obvious areas which would make Peter's COPD worse, principally smoking and being overweight. He has been told that changes to his lifestyle such as a healthier diet, gentle exercise and reducing his smoking would make a huge difference to his health, but it does not make a difference to his behaviour.

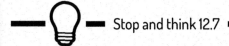 **Stop and think 12.7**

Why do some patients make lifestyle changes and others do not?

Many people feel there are too many barriers to making changes and focus only on the negative aspects of behaviour change rather than the benefits. This results in **ambivalence to change**. Instead of viewing the patient as an individual who does not want to change, MI is concerned with focusing on what the patient wants and how to achieve that goal. It is selectively eliciting and reinforcing the patient's own arguments for change. It therefore encourages 'change talk' – the benefits of changing behaviour or the costs of not changing. Three core communication skills central to MI are:

1 Asking: what are the patient's goals? Get to know them and develop a relationship with the person.
2 Informing: give the patient options and check their understanding.
3 Listening: respect the patient's wishes and offer help appropriately.

The communication skills used in MI are, for example, making summaries, reflective listening both to show empathy and lead patients to 'change talk', and using open questions. Use of open questions and reflection avoids the question-and-answer dialogue associated with closed questions that can often restrict communication between health professionals and the patient. It also avoids the 'righting reflex' whereby a nurse tries to fix things through information or advice and getting into a confrontative argument with the patient. In motivational interviewing **'rolling with resistance'** is better, by accepting that behaviour change is generated by the patient and not the health professional.

MI is not a technique or tool but a clinical skill grounded in an interpersonal relationship with the patient; it derives from a humanistic approach. It is a guiding style for developing intrinsic motivation to change (Rollnick et al., 2008). The important principles can be described by the acronym RULE:

- resist the righting reflex
- understand your patient's motivations
- listen to your patient
- empower your patient.

The evidence for MI is predominantly in the treatment of drug and alcohol misuse but since it has been applied within general healthcare it is increasingly becoming more popular, for example, in smoking cessation (Lindson-Hawley et al., 2015) or self-care in heart failure (Riegel et al., 2017).

Knowledge link You will find more detail on behaviour change and applying motivational interviewing in Chapter 15.

Conclusion

This chapter encourages you as a nurse to consider the communication issues prevalent in supporting patients living with chronic illness. It highlights the need to work, non-judgementally, with patients' own motivations in changing behaviour. This is applicable when working in either an acute or community-based environment. It also identifies difficult areas in communication such as working with patients who have received significant news and issues of bereavement and loss. One of the key aspects of communication is to identify patients' concerns. Patients living with chronic illness or disability are 'experts' in living with many competing health issues. Nurses need to take seriously the patient's own narrative in how to cope with ill health and how to support them when accessing and receiving healthcare.

FURTHER READING

Andrews, J. (2015) *Dementia: The One-stop Guide: Practical Advice for Families, Professionals and People Living with Dementia and Alzheimer's Disease.* London, Profile Books.

Kissane, D.W., Bultz, B.D., Butow, P.N., Byland, C.L., Noble, S. and Wilkinson, S. (2018) *Oxford Textbook of Communication in Oncology and Palliative Care.* Oxford, Oxford University Press.

Motschnig, R. and Nykl, L. (2014) *Person-centred Communication: Theory, Skills and Practice.* Maidenhead, Open University Press.

Rosengren, D.B. (2017) *Building Motivational Interviewing Skills: A Practical Workbook (Application of Motivating Interviewing)* (2nd edn). New York, The Guilford Press.

REFERENCES

Boss, P. (1999) *Ambiguous Loss.* Cambridge, MA, Havard University Press.

Bowlby, J. and Parkes, C.M. (1970) Separation and loss within the family. In E.J. Anthony and C. Koupernik (eds), *The Child in his Family* (pp. 197–216). Wiley, Chichester.

Butow, P.N., Brown, R.F., Cogar, S., Tattersall, M.H. and Dunn, S.M. (2002) Oncologists' reactions to cancer patients' verbal cues. *Psycho-oncology*, 11, 47–58.

Delgado, C., Upton, D., Ranse, K., Furness, T. and Foster, K. (2017) Nurses' resilience and the emotional labour of nursing work: an integrative review of empirical literature. *International Journal of Nursing Studies*, 70, 71–88.

Del Piccolo, L., Goss, C. and Bergvik, S. (2006) The fourth meeting of the Verona network on sequence analysis 'consensus finding on the appropriateness of provider responses to patient cues and concerns'. *Patient Education and Counseling*, 60, 313–325.

Department of Health (2005) *National Service Framework for Long-term Conditions.* www.dh.gov.uk/en/Publicationsandstatistics/Publications/PublicationsPolicyAndGuidance/DH_4105361.

Department of Health (2006) *Our Health, Our Care, Our Say: A New Direction for Community Services.* London, Department of Health Publications.

Department of Health (2008) *End of Life Care Strategy.* London, Department of Health.

Department of Health (2010) *Improving the Health and Wellbeing of People with Long-term Conditions. World Class Services for People with Long-term Conditions: Information Tool for Commissioners*. London, Department of Health Publications.

Department of Health (2012) *Long-term Conditions Compendium of Information* (3rd edn). www.gov.uk/government/publications/long-term-conditions-compendium-of-information-third-edition.

Department of Health (2014) *Five Year Forward View*. www.england.nhs.uk/wp-content/uploads/2014/10/5yfv-web.pdf.

Didion, J. (2005) *The Year of Magical Thinking*. London, Fourth Estate.

Duncan, M., Moschopoulou, E., Herrington, E., Deane, J., Raglance, R., Jones, L., Bourke, L., Morgan, A., Chalder, T., Thaha, M., Taylor, S., Korszun, A., White, P. and Bhui, K. (2017) Review of systematic reviews of non-pharmacological interventions to improve quality of life in cancer survivors. *BMJ Open*, 7, e015860.

Friedrichsen, M. and Milberg, A. (2006) Concerns about losing control when breaking bad news to terminally ill patients with cancer: physician's perspective. *Journal of Palliative Medicine*, 9, 673–682.

Goodwin, N., Curry, N., Naylor, C., Ross, S. and Duldig, W. (2010) *Managing People with Long-term Conditions*. The King's Fund. www.kingsfund.org.uk/sites/default/files/field/field_document/managing-people-long-term-conditions-gp-inquiry-research-paper-mar11.pdf.

Gorawara-Bhat, R., Hafskjold, L., Gulbrandsen, P. and Eide, H. (2017) Exploring physicians' verbal and non-verbal responses to cues/concerns: learning from incongruent communication. *Patient Education and Counseling*, 100(11), 1979–1989.

Hind, D., Cotter, J., Thake, A., Bradburn, M., Cooper, C., Isaac, C. and House, A. (2014) Cognitive behavioural theory for the treatment of depression in people with multiple sclerosis: a systematic review and meta-analysis. *BMC Psychiatry*, 14(5). doi: 10.1186/1471-244x-14-5.

Holdsworth, L.M. (2015) Bereaved carers' accounts of the end of life and the role of care providers in a 'good death': a qualitative study. *Palliative Medicine*, 29(9), 834–841.

Kingston, A., Comas-Herrera, A. and Jagger, C. (2018) Forecasting the care needs of the older population in England over the next 20 years: estimates from the Population Ageing and Care Simulation (PACSIM) modelling study. *The Lancet: Public Health*, 3(9), PE447–PE455.

Kruijver, I., Kerkstra, A., Bensing, J. and van de Weil, H. (2001) Communication skills for nurses during interactions with simulated cancer patients. *Journal of Advanced Nursing*, 34(6), 772–779.

Kubler-Ross, E. (1970) *On Death and Dying*. London, Tavistock.

Lindson-Hawley, N., Thompson, T.P. and Begh, R. (2015) Motivational interviewing for smoking cessation. *Cochrane Database of Systematic Reviews*, 3, CD006936.

Mallon, B. (2008) *Dying, Death and Grief: Working with Adult Bereavement*. London, SAGE Publications.

Miller, W.R. and Rollnick, S. (2002) *Motivational Interviewing* (2nd edn). New York, The Guilford Press.

Ostelo, R., van Tulder, M., Vlaeyens, J., Linton, S., Morley, S. and Assendelft, W. (2005) Behavioural treatment for chronic back pain. *Cochrane Database of Systematic Reviews*, 1, CD002104.

PHE (2018) *Health Profile for England: The Health of England Today and into the Future*. https://publichealthmatters.blog.gov.uk/2018/09/11/health-profile-for-england-the-health-of-england-today-and-into-the-future/.

Riegel, B., Dickson, V.V., Garcia, L.E., Creber, R.M. and Streur, M. (2017) Mechanisms of change in self-care in adults with heart failure receiving a tailored, motivational interviewing intervention. *Patient Education and Counseling*, 100(2), 283–288.

Rollnick, S., Miller, W. and Butler, C. (2008) *Motivational Interviewing in Healthcare*. New York, The Guilford Press.

Shaw, J., Brown, R. and, Dunn, S. (2015) The impact of delivery style on doctors' experience of stress during simulated bad news consultations. *Patient Education and Counseling*, 98(10), 1255–1259.

Spiegel, W., Thomas, Z., Maier, M., Vutuc, C., Isak, K., Karlic, H. and Michsche, M. (2009) Breaking bad news to cancer patients: survey & analysis. *Psycho-Oncology*, 18(2), 179–186.

Tully, P., Selkow, T., Bengel, J. and Rafanelli, C. (2015) A dynamic view of comorbid depression and generalized anxiety disorder symptom change in chronic heart failure: the discrete effects of cognitive behavioral therapy, exercise, and psychotropic medication. *Disability and Rehabilitation*, 37(7), 585–592.

Vos, M. and de Haes, J. (2007) Denial in cancer patients, an explorative review. *Psycho-Oncology*, 16, 12–25.

Walter, T. (1996) A new model of grief: bereavement and biography. *Mortality*, 1(1), 7–25.

WHO (2018) *Fact Sheets: Ageing and health*. World Health Organization. www.who.int/news-room/fact-sheets/detail/ageing-and-health.

Wittenberg-Lyles, E., Goldsmith, J., Sanchez-Reilly, S. and Ragan, S. (2008) Communicating a terminal prognosis in a palliative care setting: deficiencies in current communication training protocols. *Social Science and Medicine*, 66, 2356–2365.

Worden, J.W. (1991) *Grief Counselling and Grief Therapy: A Handbook for the Mental Health Practitioner* (2nd edn). London, Routledge.

Ye, M., Du, K., Zhohu, J., Zhou, Q., Shou, M., Hu, B., Jiang, P., Dong, N., He, L., Liang, S., Yu, C., Zhang, J., Ding, Z. and Liu, Z. (2018) A meta-analysis of the efficacy of cognitive behaviour therapy on quality of life and psychological health of breast cancer survivors and patients. *Psycho-Oncology*, 27(7), 1695–1703.

Zwingmann, J., Baile, W.F., Schmier, J.W., Bernhard, J. and Keller, M. (2017) Effects of patient-centred communication on anxiety, negative affect and trust in the physician in delivering a cancer diagnosis: a randomized, experimental study. *Cancer*, 123(16), 3167–3175.

THIRTEEN
COMMUNICATING WITH CHILDREN, YOUNG PEOPLE AND THEIR FAMILIES
CAROLINE RIDLEY

.... THIS CHAPTER WILL HELP YOU TO:

- Communicate effectively and sensitively with children, young people and their families in different settings, using a range of methods and skills
- Appreciate different cultural traditions, beliefs, UK legal frameworks and professional ethics
- Be proactive and creative in enhancing communication and understanding
- Act professionally and autonomously in situations when needing to take safeguarding into account
- Provide safe and effective care in partnership in the context of people's ages, conditions and developmental stages
- Make effective referrals to safeguard and protect children and adults requiring support and protection
- Work with people to provide clear and accurate information

Introduction

All health professionals will have contact with children and young people and all have a duty of care to ensure their safety across the range of settings in which they work. A young person may be an informal carer, or dependent on the care of someone with a serious mental, physical or behavioural disability. Similarly, children and young people are encountered in clinical areas as patients, dependants and visitors.

The variety of ways children and young people live, learn and play, and the transition into different types of family groups for many children, creates new challenges and opportunities. Nursing the child frequently means nursing the family as the needs of children are inextricably linked to the needs of their carers. Communication with these users of healthcare services is not always straightforward and involves nurses in both acute and primary care settings being willing and able to listen, explain, empower, consult and negotiate, empathise, challenge, reward and stimulate (Department for Education and Skills (DfES), 2004). Although some of these skills and related issues are discussed more specifically in particular sections of this chapter, they are transferable skills that can be equally applied across the other areas described.

Getting involved

Nurses working in specialist fields of child health are ideally placed to meet their complex needs. However, *all* nurses have a duty of care to provide general care and to recognise difficulties early, make timely and appropriate referrals to other agencies and encourage, promote and support optimum health (DfES, 2004). To do this successfully, nurses need to have a basic knowledge of child development and an understanding of the risk factors that can lead to health breakdown. Developing a confident working knowledge in these areas will serve to ensure any communication you have with children and young people is productive and in their best interests.

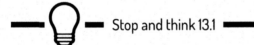 Stop and think 13.1

Consider the different communication needs of children and young people in the following age groups:

infant

toddler

pre-school

primary school

adolescent.

Think of the different ways a nurse may communicate effectively with these different age groups. Possible answers are suggested in Table 13.1.

Table 13.1   Suggested communication styles for different age groups of children

Age of child	Types of communication
Infant	Touch, facial expression, singing, making baby faces, vocalising
Toddler	Simple language, touch, physical role-modelling and demonstrating, enactment
Pre-school age	Verbal, picture books, play modelling and enactment, cartoons, video
Primary school age	Verbal, pictures, diagrams, written (simple), video, complex physical role-modelling and enactment
Adolescent	Verbal, written, blogging, social media, texting, e-mail, leaflets, books, websites

Inclusive communication with children and young people

Communicating effectively

Effective communication with children and young people requires nurses who are pre-pared to build empathy, work in partnership and demonstrate common core skills and knowledge of issues including confidentiality, ethics and respect (DfES, 2005). According to the Department of Health's National Framework for Children, children and young people are not always treated with sensitivity or courtesy and have rights that are not always understood or respected (Department of Health, 2003). The nurses' professional code calls for nurses to 'listen to people and respond to their preferences and concerns' (NMC, 2018), yet young people themselves have identified a range of barriers to effective use of services including a lack of information and expertise as well as a failure by health professionals to respect their views (RCN, 2009). The National Children's Bureau Public Health Reference Group (Brady, 2008) emphasised the importance to young people of professionals listening to their views and not just doing it because it 'looks good', and the consultation paper *Youth Matters* also highlighted young people's desire to be heard:

> People should listen to us more. They never do, they always do what they want anyway.
>
> (DfES, 2006:13)

See Box 13.1 for an example of active listening in practice.

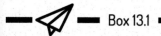 Box 13.1

Active listening in the emergency department

During a hospital assessment with a 15-year-old girl, accompanied by her father, the doctor got negative answers to the 'have you ever smoked?' and 'have you had a drink?' questions. Once her

(Continued)

father went to get some coffee, the doctor explained to the girl that the questions aimed to assess the risk to the patient and were not a judgement on her character. The doctor explained that such a history would indicate the need for thrombo-embolic deterrent (TED) stockings in surgery to avoid thrombosis. When asked again, the girl gave a history of smoking and heavy drinking.

Creative communication

Motivated nurses might consider how information technology and the use of other 'new media' communication tools could be used to enhance discourse and contact with children and young people. Digital TV, social media and widespread internet access have changed the ways in which children and young people live and learn. Almost a quarter of 8–11-year-old children and three-quarters of 12–15-year-old children have a social media profile (Ofcom, 2017), but the sites children and young people are using are frequently changing. The popularity in all childhood age groups of YouTube as a source of information and entertainment is growing and smartphone/tablet ownership, which begins in very early childhood, rises to 83% in the 12–15-year age group (Ofcom, 2017).

New technologies bring both challenges and opportunities and health-related risks such as online addiction, grooming and cyberbullying should not be underestimated. Fifteen per cent of 15 year olds reported experiencing cyberbullying in the past 2 months (Association of Young People's Health, 2017). In addition, Hinduja and Patchin (2010) reported results from a survey given to approximately 2000 middle-school children in the USA indicating that victims of cyberbullying were almost twice as likely to attempt suicide than those who had not experienced cyberbullying. However, positive effects of new media technologies offering platforms for health interventions that are particularly suitable for young people have been identified (Layard and Hagell, 2015); for instance, social media opens the door for children and young people to be more connected with family and friends, be more active within their communities and have better access to health information (Royal Society of Public Health, 2017). Using social media, nurses and other care staff can share information and gather feedback from children and young people about what they want and need. Text messaging services such as appointment reminders, responses to requests about services and personalised health advice are all being used effectively across different Trusts and partnerships, and guidance from the RCN (2014) provides useful information for nurses who might want to use text messaging when working with children and young people.

Traditional forms of written communication may impede those with restricted physical access or reading from full and meaningful engagement. Dyslexia can remain a hidden disability but is believed to affect around 10% of the population, and 4% severely so (British Dyslexia Association, 2018). These particular children and young people might benefit from alternative ways of communicating such as those with an increased emphasis on visual imagery. Try to give children and young people with attention-deficit hyperactivity disorder (ADHD) individual attention in a relaxed environment. Communicate with them on a one-to-one basis and avoid talking to other children at the same time. Children or young people with autism spectrum disorder will present with varying degrees of communication difficulty but a common problem across the spectrum is their difficulty relating to others. Be aware of your non-verbal signals such as posture, facial expression pitch and tone of voice.

Electronically mailed information means children and young people can access it at a time and place suited to them and in a way specifically suited to their particular learning needs. Those who use only non-verbal communication might require interpreters or signers to ensure full participation in any consultation and those with learning/behavioural difficulties such as autism and ADHD may benefit from the inclusion of their family, primary carers or advocacy services.

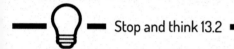 Stop and think 13.2

Not all children or young people with a hidden communication difficulty such as dyslexia will choose to disclose their disability to you. What strategies might you employ that would optimise any contact these children and young people have with you and your service? The answer is inclusive communication, as outlined below.

a   Spend time getting to know the child or young person. Making time reflects your interest in them and makes it more likely that they will share any difficulties with you. Reassure them about confidentiality.
b   Be proactive. Do not be afraid to ask direct questions such as 'do you have any particular preferences regarding communication? Would it be easier for me to write to you with future appointments or to call or text you?'
c   Support written information with verbal/visual/practical explanations. Avoid jargon or complex language. Ask the child or young person if they would like anyone to be present during your consultation.
d   Create an atmosphere that facilitates disclosure. A poster on the wall about dyslexia, for example, may signal your department's recognition of the condition. It is legitimate to refer to 'some other' children and young people who have told you they have had difficulty reading information given to them. This may reduce any feelings of isolation.

Fraser guidelines and Gillick competence

Age may be a determinant in assessing a child or young person's competence but it is not always a reliable indicator of their ability to make informed and independent decisions regarding health advice and treatment. The Fraser guidelines (NSPCC, 2018) support the objective assessment of an individual's level of competence relating to contraceptive advice and treatment (Gillick v West Norfolk and Wisbech AHA, 1985), but the test for so-called 'Gillick competence' has been more widely used in healthcare settings to help assess whether a child has the maturity to make their own decisions and to understand the implications of those decisions in relation to a range of healthcare choices (NSPCC, 2018). Children under 16 may be deemed Gillick-competent if they are able to:

- understand the reasons for and nature of any treatment that is offered
- understand the principal benefits and risks of treatment and available alternative courses of action
- understand the consequences of any refusal to have treatment
- be able to make a choice free from coercion or pressure.

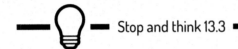 Stop and think 13.3

Consider an occasion in your own practice where the test for Gillick competence might be applied. What questions would you need to ask the child or young person and how would you document the consultation? Who within the multi-professional team might you need to consult with to deliver the best possible care for your patient?

Suggested answer: assessment of Gillick competence:

a   Explain issues clearly, free from unnecessary jargon. Make time for questions and consideration of the issues before they make their decision. Suitable questions to ask may include inviting the child or young person to repeat instructions for taking medication, asking them to tell you what might happen if they do not comply with the preferred choice of treatment and to tell you about any possible side effects of treatment.

b   You should document clearly in writing what you have discussed with your patient including reference to the questions you have asked and the child/young person's responses. For example, 'the young person was able to describe the condition and reason for treatment' (RCN, 2013:12).

c   Liaison with other professionals caring for the patient such as a paediatrician, teacher or social worker will help you make a well-informed decision. Any consultations should be recorded with details of what was agreed and by whom.

Communicating with children/young people at home

The environment is an important factor in shaping communication (Hargie and Dickson, 2004) and, in 2001, the Department of Health (2001) was calling for children's and young people's healthcare and treatment to be delivered in settings that cause minimal disruption to their ordinary home life. In the home setting the balance of power between professional and patient means children and young people may feel less threatened and more able to talk honestly and openly about matters of importance to them (Shaw, 2009).

Trust between the nurse and patient is built by a commitment to respect an individual's cultural norms and values. At home the unique ways in which a child or young person and their family live can be open to scrutiny and judgement. Engagement with children and young people requires a degree of humility and nurses have to learn to accept that others' values and beliefs are as valid and important as theirs are to themselves (Hugman, 2009).

> Many people have a natural prejudice in favour of their own cultural heritage and upbringing.
>
> (Hugman, 2009:128)

Young carers

Nurses working with children or young people at home should be mindful of those young carers looking after family members at home. While community nurses are more likely to be involved with families where a member has a long-term illness, many children who are carers remain hidden in the community, fearful of professional intervention that may threaten their home life and routine (Aldridge and Becker, 1993). Department of Health (2008) guidance reminds healthcare professionals of the detrimental effects caring can have on young carers' physical and emotional health and has called for whole family support in these circumstances. Box 13.2 lists some practical ways in which you might communicate effectively with young carers.

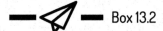 Box 13.2

Dealing with young carers

- Be alert to children or young people who are carers and approach the issue with sensitivity and understanding.
- Encourage young carers to talk to you about their responsibilities so that appropriate support packages might be employed. Children and young people may need to be told that they have a choice about taking on a caring role.
- Every young carer's situation is unique. Listen to what the young carer wants or needs. With their permission, make referrals to other agencies as necessary.
- Encourage young carers to engage with opportunities to enhance their own health and wellbeing.

(Continued)

- Children should not be used as interpreters in health settings as it places them in a difficult and prematurely adult role (British Psychological Society, 2017). In the family home this may be unavoidable, however, it is important to remind families that a professional interpreter can be made available to them and to familiarise yourself with local arrangements.
- Keep lines of communication open. When your role with the family ends, take steps to ensure the young person is in contact with others who can help, such as Connexions, the local young carers forum or charitable organisations such as The Children's Society.

Methods of communication in community settings

A home visit may be the first time a nurse and child or young person meet, and how the initial contact is made to arrange the meeting can affect the ensuing relationship. Warmth and friendliness can be conveyed through the language you use in a text message, a letter or phone call, and the tone of your voice might help to break down a perception of the nurse as authoritative and interfering rather than empowering and supportive. Letters to children or young people may be opened by adults with or without parental responsibility and not everyone can read well. A telephone call or text message may be more appropriate. Might you be introduced via a colleague already working with the child or young person and whose trust is established? Remember, families may be apprehensive at the thought of your visit, especially if you are calling because of challenging issues such as teenage pregnancy or suggested abuse.

Once a mutually convenient appointment has been arranged it is useful to ask yourself the following questions before your visit:

- Is the visit really necessary? Time is a valuable resource and should not be abused or wasted.
- Is the purpose of your visit clear? Do you have enough background information to guide your planning and determine clear aims and objectives?
- Where can you obtain appropriate and necessary background information? Remember to follow the procedures and legislation related to matters of confidentiality for your particular job role. There should be no 'hidden agenda' and the child or young person and their carers should feel equally prepared and ready for your visit.
- How old is the child or young person you are visiting? Failure to address different levels of maturity between children can undermine the nurse's attempt to form a rapport (Thompson, 2009). Can the child or young person communicate effectively themselves or is the nurse reliant on information from the parent or carer? Wherever possible, communicate directly with the child or young person even if they are relatively young (Berry, 2007). What difference will this make to your planning? Will you need, for example, to request a private space to facilitate a young person's right to confidential advice and treatment?

- Have you considered the impact of the family dynamics? Parents or carers should usually be expected to know their children best (DfES, 2004) but family tension and relationship complexities will influence any communication you have with your patient. For example, a child who is fearful of their parent may remain silent and withdraw from the consultation. Younger teenagers may want their parents involved but older teenagers may not (Berry, 2007). The observant nurse will be attuned to non-verbal signals that offer clues about how a child or young person might really be feeling. See Practice example box 13.1. It is important that you record information accurately to support patient care and communications (NMC, 2018).
- What is the relationship between the carer and the child or young person? Observe eye contact between the child or young person and their carer. Do they seem anxious and too willing to please? Are they checking that their responses are met with approval? Do they contribute freely to the conversation or are they more restrained?
- Who has parental responsibility and who should be involved in the consultation and kept informed? In the child or young person's home you will have less control over the physical environment and you may need to exercise negotiation skills in order to request that particular individuals leave the room, or make a polite request that interruptions to your consultation are minimised.

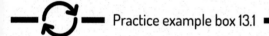 **Practice example box 13.1**

Reading non-verbal communication

A family consisting of both parents, two boys (aged 12 and 8) and an older girl (aged 14) had been convened for a family therapy session. The discussion between the parents and the older boy became quite heated and it was noted that the younger boy then went to look out of the window. In doing so, he had created a barrier of the backs of the chairs between himself and the heated discussion. This was a significant indicator to his own distress at the family's problems, but he was not empowered to express this distress openly.

Knowledge link See Chapter 8 for more on overcoming communication difficulties in the home visit.

Communicating with the child or young person in hospital

The environment as a barrier

A hospital can be a strange place to a child or young person. There are staff in uniform, unusual smells, unfamiliar noises, scary medical equipment and an unfamiliar cot or bed.

All of these may precipitate stress, anxiety and fear. Nurses working in hospital settings are ideally placed to consider the environment in which they work. Creating an atmosphere of warmth and friendliness on a ward or clinic may seem obvious, but communication is further enhanced through less obvious measures such as low reception desks so children can see the faces of staff involved in their care, easy wheelchair/pushchair access, clear signposting and provision of private areas for those in need (NHS Estates, 2003).

Family–centred care

Promoted as an ideal model of care for meeting the needs of hospitalised children and young people, Shields et al. (2006) define family-centred care as:

> a way of caring for children and their families within health services which ensures that care is planned around the whole family, not just the individual child/person and in which all the family members are recognised as care recipients.
>
> (Shields et al., 2006:1318)

This fits well with Children's Hospital Standard (Department of Health, 2003) that makes explicit reference to a need for hospital services to be centred around the needs of children and their families. The Bristol Royal Infirmary Inquiry (COI Communications, 2001) found that hospital facilities frequently failed to address the differing needs of children and young people at different ages, treating them all as 'mini adults' rather than discrete groups with particular and specific needs. Children who are frightened by pain or illness may be further disadvantaged by having to communicate their concerns to strangers (Elliott, 2009). Staff working in hospitals must be willing to listen to children and young people and provide information that is factual, objective and non-directive (Department of Health, 2003). Evidence has revealed that children are more compliant and better able to endure treatment if they have been involved in decision-making and empowered to retain a sense of control over the situation (Runeson, 2002). Sick children and young people have a compelling desire for health professionals to give them honest, clear and in-depth information (Smith and Callery, 2005). In Young et al.'s (2003) study of communication about cancer in childhood, parents found that communication with their children became more honest and open as parents became less 'controlling' and communicated more as 'partners' as the illness and treatment progressed.

Managing complex communication

Nurses utilising active listening skills will be attuned to non-verbal and verbal signals that offer clues to a child or young person's readiness to engage in conversation.

Asking questions of you may indicate their interest or concern. Eye contact may be a clue to a child's desire to be heard, and defensive body language may suggest tension or fear. See Practice example box 13.2 for an example of active listening skills in practice.

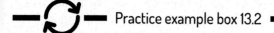 Practice example box 13.2

Active listening skills on a medical ward

A shy teenage girl's frequent vomiting was puzzling everyone on the medical team. Major medical and behavioural factors had been ruled out. Having resolved to give up and discharge her, a junior doctor asked her if there was anything the girl wished someone had asked her during her stay in hospital. The girl replied that she had recently lost her grandmother who she was very fond of, but nobody had asked her to talk about things like that.

Knowledge link See Chapter 4 for detailed explanation of active listening skills.

Children and young people may commonly use euphemisms or 'slang' language to describe their feelings, their conditions or problems and when referring to body parts. They may feel more relaxed using their own language particularly if the issue they are discussing is embarrassing or highly personal. While it is important to communicate with them in a way they understand, it is also important that you, as the health professional, seek clarification over language you are unfamiliar with or simply do not know.

Communicating through play

Play is a fundamental aspect of healthy childhood. Play provides valuable information about a child's cognitive development and language ability and can be helpful in conveying information, facilitating questions as well as helping children express fears and anxieties. Play can help children regain confidence and self-esteem, understand illness and treatment and supports a speedier recovery (National Association of Health Play Specialists, 2018). Mathisen and Butterworth (2001) refer to three forms of play, all of which require skilled communication to engage the child, as follows.

1 *Normative* or *everyday play* in hospital helps recreate the familiar, serves to distract children and enhances feelings of security.
2 *Educative play* enables the transfer of information to the child.

3   *Therapeutic play* can be used to help children make sense of their illness and may support better understanding of a procedure or treatment.

Activities normally enjoyed by children when they are well can often be adapted for situations when they are unwell, and finding activities they can enjoy helps normalise a situation and demonstrates a nurse's interest in and care for them (Elliott, 2009). Play should be age-appropriate and a range of activities should be considered:

Babies enjoy toys that serve to engage and distract, such as mobiles and colourful visual imagery. The use of music may be comforting. The tone and pitch of the nurse's voice will impact on a baby's behaviour and emotional state.

Toddlers can be strong willed as they develop their 'sense of self'. Toddlers respond to nurses who are patient, friendly and willing to engage and explain. Through the use of dolls and teddies a nurse can demonstrate a procedure and help the toddler 'see' and 'feel' what might happen. The nurse can observe the toddler's reaction to better understand their concerns. Toddlers are sensitive to both verbal and non-verbal cues and are attuned to their surroundings so the effect of a nurse's language and behaviour towards both the toddler and their family should be considered.

Pre-school children can express their feelings through drawing and painting. They are often sociable and friendly. Imaginative and 'pretend' play may offer clues to what they are feeling (Dunn, 2004). Educative play through the use of stories, for example, can help the pre-school child better understand what will happen. It is important to build trust, and nurses must be honest when explaining any procedures or treatments (Sepion, 2009). The nurse–young patient relationship can trigger pertinent questions and strengthen professional bonds.

Primary-aged children in hospital should be invited to engage with health professionals about what is going to happen. They are usually able to articulate their needs well. School-aged children can answer questions and have the right to be included in conversations about their illness and treatment. Writing poems, verses and cards can also provide insight into a child's thoughts and facilitate communication with those they care most about.

Knowledge link Further useful information and guidance for staff can be found in guidance from the National Association of Health Play Specialists (2018) (www.nahps.org.uk/publications/).

How young people want to be communicated with

Young people in hospital require careful consideration. When interviewed in Kelsey and Abelson-Mitchell's (2007) study exploring their perceptions of their involvement in healthcare, respondents reported satisfactory experiences when staff exercised the following communication traits:

- speaking directly to them when seeking relevant information
- accommodating their specific needs, thereby demonstrating listening skills, support and attention
- making sure language was understandable and avoiding technical jargon
- making them feel comfortable and being kind and empathetic.

Poor experiences were associated with the following communication traits and triggered feelings including frustration, worry and lack of trust:

- not focusing on *them*; for example the professional speaking directly to a parent
- emphasising the power difference through behaviours such as 'siding' with parents or asking questions they were not able to understand
- not being honest
- demonstrating through non-verbal signals a lack of interest in them such as looking at notes during a consultation.

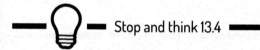 Stop and think 13.4

The transition from child to adult services can be challenging for young people with long-term conditions such as arthritis. Consider communication strategies that might alleviate stress and anxiety at this time.

Suggested answer: transition from child to adult services:

a   Find out the young person's concerns. The parents could also be asked this.
b   With the young person and parents, work out questions that will need to be answered. Do this separately with the child and the parents. Suggest to the young person that they rehearse with you or their parents what they want to say to or ask of the adult team so that they become more confident in their communication with someone they know first.
c   Arrange a personal introduction and visit to adult services. Plan with the young person when they will meet the adult team with their parents, and without their parents and with a friend. Provide a list of key professionals in both child and adult services who may be contacted if problems arise.
d   Plan with the young person to start taking on more responsibilities for self-care and self-medication.
e   Suggest to the young person that they keep a diary in which they can record their self-care, unexpected issues and feelings.

Engagement with parents and siblings in hospital

Parental anxiety due to the hospitalisation of a child may serve to decrease the amount of involvement that some parents feel able to commit to in caring for their sick child

(Coyne, 1994). Parents are usually the experts on their child yet they may feel disempowered in the hospital setting, which increases their own anxiety. Evidence demonstrates that parents often feel excluded from the decision-making processes (Hummelinck and Pollock, 2006) and report feeling anxious when observed by nurses (Darbyshire, 1994). While older children may have different wishes to those of their parents, skilled nurses will be mindful of the need to support both parties if optimum outcomes for the child or young person are to prevail. Being approachable with a willingness to answer questions and making time to talk with parents are important and nurses should be alert to the misunderstandings that can originate from the use of medical jargon.

Family-centred care attends to the needs and influence of siblings. Craft and Craft (1989) and O'Shea et al. (2012) found siblings of sick children were often neglected and it is easy for the needs of a very ill child to dominate the thoughts of parents in a way that ignores the less pressing needs of a well brother or sister. Appropriate and thoughtful explanation to a sibling can facilitate positive outcomes for all children in the family (see Box 13.3).

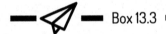 Box 13.3

Family-centred care in health visiting

A mother is preoccupied with her 6-week-old baby who has persistent colic. She is breastfeeding and still recovering from a complicated labour and birth. Her toddler son is confused and upset at the change of circumstances at home and missing the attention he normally gets from his mother. He associates crying and screaming with the receipt of affection and begins throwing violent temper tantrums. When his mother acknowledges his feelings, includes him in the care of the baby and makes time to play/read/eat/rest with him during quieter moments in the day, his behaviour improves and the family are more relaxed.

Visit the Great Ormond Street Hospital website and see their advice to parents when managing a sibling of a child in hospital (www.gosh.nhs.uk/parents-and-visitors/advice-when-you-stay/coping-hospital-visit/helping-your-other-children-cope).

The vulnerable child or young person

Knowing what the child or young person expects from any interaction you have with them is important, as is your responsibility to explain your role and any limitations clearly. This is particularly important when children and young people are considering disclosing sensitive or highly personal information such as abuse. Particular groups of children and young people have been identified as more susceptible to poorer health outcomes and more in need of professionals' heightened awareness (Department of Health,

2004). This includes those experiencing psychological or social disadvantage, looked-after children and those with family care responsibilities. *Future in Mind* (Department of Health, 2015) reported that one in 10 children need support for mental health problems, and those affected by mental ill health are likely to have a range of needs requiring assistance or intervention. Some nurses, such as school nurses and health visitors, work closely with children and young people with psychological difficulties. While it may be more natural to adopt a parental approach due to age difference (Machin and Watson, 2018), an approach that is inclusive, non-judgemental, supportive and hopeful may work best. Vulnerable children and young people may be less able to approach health professionals and it is vital that nurses do not miss valuable opportunities for contact. Recognising potential communication barriers and responding in a timely and appropriate manner increases the likelihood of improved health outcomes and a positive relationship with health professionals.

Communication barriers

Whether you are in a child or adult placement setting, Table 13.2 shows a brief checklist to help you consider how you can reduce potential communication barriers that might exist.

Table 13.2 A brief checklist to help reduce potential communication barriers

Communication barrier	Considerations for nurses
Uniform and appearance	• Is it really necessary? • Is it intimidating? • Is the nurse distinctly recognisable? • If you are wearing regular clothing is your status/name clearly visible? • Are you carrying your personal medical equipment, e.g. a stethoscope?
Administrative systems	• Do you have a formal appointment system? Can you be more flexible? • How about drop-in centres located within schools, colleges and the community?
Demeanour	• Are you interested, approachable and friendly? Have you said hello? • Have you used the patient's preferred name? • Have you introduced yourself? • Do you look as if you have time to listen? • Are you prepared to drop everything for an important disclosure? Never underestimate the courage it takes for children and young people to come forward. This might be your only chance to offer support.
Non-verbal signals	• Eye contact; an important channel of communication, demonstrates warmth, interest and concern and builds trust. • Do you smile? It helps break down barriers and builds trust. • Posture. The way you walk, stand and sit conveys powerful messages.

(Continued)

Table 13.2 (Continued)

Communication barrier	Considerations for nurses
Setting	• Does the setting feel safe and welcoming?
	• Is it child- or young person-friendly?
	• Do you have a suggestions/comment box?
Verbal communication	• Think about the language you use. Do you avoid technical/medical jargon?
	• How do you check the information you give is understood? Asking the child/young person to repeat information is a simple way to check understanding.
	• How clearly do you speak? The success of verbal communication is influenced by the tone, pitch and rhythm of your voice.
	• What if you don't know something? It is better to be honest and invite the young person to speak to someone else or for you to find out on their behalf.
Confidentiality policies and guidelines	• Do you have a confidentiality policy that reflects professional and legislative practice and guidance? Absolute confidentiality cannot always be guaranteed and if you believe there is a risk to the health, safety or welfare of a child or young person then that matter is serious enough to outweigh the patient's right to privacy.
	• In all other circumstances, nurses are duty bound to uphold a child or young person's right to confidential advice and treatment.
	• Children and young people want clarity about confidentiality procedures. Is your confidentiality policy clearly stated and prominently placed in your workplace?

The teenage parent

Young parents have been identified as a particularly vulnerable group. They endure poorer child health outcomes, poorer emotional health and wellbeing and poorer economic wellbeing compared with older parents (PHE, 2015). Young parents have spoken of healthcare professionals who are sometimes judgemental and unresponsive to their particular needs, making them less likely to attend for antenatal care (DCSF/DH, 2007). They have reported feeling 'singled out' and 'being checked up on', and young fathers have reported feeling unwelcome and ignored, with resultant disengagement from consultations and appointments (DCSF/DH, 2007). Young people may mistrust authority or fear being judged (PHE, 2015) and are concerned about issues relating to confidentiality and trust (Croghan et al., 2004; DCSF/DH, 2009). When first year undergraduate nursing students were asked in Leishman's (2004) study what might reduce the *risk* of teenage pregnancy, responses included:

• not being judgemental
• not telling off young people or talking down to them when they seek advice
• being an educator and providing information at an appropriate level that can easily be understood.

These thoughts are mirrored elsewhere (DfES, 2006) and the list below offers further information to support you when working with teenage parents:

1   Show them respect. Teenage parents can be confident, capable and caring. Respectful communication includes not making assumptions or relying on stereotypes (Thompson, 2009).
2   Listen actively. Listen carefully to what they have to say. Paraphrasing helps establish empathy and provides an opportunity for the young person to confirm or adjust what they have said (Moss, 2008).
3   Observe carefully. Uncommunicative teenage parents may give clues to their emotional state through non-verbal language such as poor eye contact or busying themselves with their child during a consultation. Offer more time and use closed questions to reduce their stress and anxiety (Lloyd and Bor, 2004).
4   Be non-judgemental. Avoid making assumptions about their situation or behaviour.
5   Empower. Empowered teenage parents are enabled to make appropriate decisions and take responsibility for their own actions. Avoid fault-finding and be 'open, positive, empathic and supportive' (De Vito, 2009:300).
6   Respect confidentiality. *You're Welcome Pilot* quality criteria (Department of Health, 2017) assist providers of healthcare services to make services friendly to young people. Teenage parents have a right to a confidential service and the principles include a need for professional teams to have a shared understanding of their confidentiality procedures, to display the policy clearly and, in line with digital health developments, explain to young people when they can access their records and their parents cannot.
7   Be flexible. Teenage parents may need to access services outside of the school, college or work setting and will respond more appropriately if they are offered flexible services and appointment times.

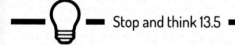 Stop and think 13.5

Go back to Stop and think 13.1. Can you now add more communication methods to your list?

Conclusion

This chapter has introduced you to the diverse communication needs of children and young people in a range of settings in which contact may be made. The health and well-being of every child and young person is important and healthcare professionals who are motivated to develop and practise skilled communication techniques will facilitate the development of meaningful relationships that address these needs, now and into the adult years.

....FURTHER READING

Burton, M., Pavod, E. and Williams, B. (2014) *An Introduction to Child and Adolescent Mental Health*. London, SAGE Publications.

Chalmers, D. (2016) *Communicating with Children from Birth to Four Years*. Oxford, Routledge.

Davies, L. and Kerrigan Lebloch, E. (2013) *Communicating with Children and their Families: Responding to Need and Protection*. Maidenhead, Open University Press.

Hubbuck, C. (2009) *Play for Sick Children: Play Specialists in Hospitals and Beyond*. London, Jessica Kingsley.

Levevre, M. (2018) *Communicating with Children and Young People: Making a Difference* (2nd edn). Bristol, Policy Press.

McDonald, J.D. (2004) *Communicating Partners: 30 Years of Building Responsive Relationships with Late Talking Children including Autism, Asperger's Syndrome (ASD), Down Syndrome, and Typical Development*. London, Jessica Kingsley.

Reid, G. (2016) *Dyslexia: A Practitioner's Handbook* (5th edn). Chichester, Wiley Blackwell.

Sheridan, M., Sharma, A. and Cockerill, H. (2014) *From Birth to Five Years: Children's Developmental Progress* (4th edn). New York, Routledge.

Smith, P. (2010) *Understanding Children's Worlds: Children and Play*. Chichester, Wiley Blackwell.

Winter, K. (2011) *Building Relationships and Communicating with Young Children: A Practical Guide for Social Workers*. Abingdon, Routledge.

....REFERENCES

Aldridge, J. and Becker, S. (1993) Children as carers. *Archives of Disease in Childhood*, 69, 459–462.

Association of Young People's Health (2017) *Key Data on Young People*. www.ayph.org.uk/keydata2017/FullVersion2017.

Berry, D. (2007) *Health Communication Theory and Practice*. Maidenhead, Open University Press.

Brady, L.M. (2008) *National Children's Bureau. Young People's Public Health Reference Group. Pilot Project-Final Report*. January 2008. www.york.ac.uk/phrc/YPPHRG_FR_1.08.pdf.

British Dyslexia Association (2018) *Dyslexia and Co-occurring Difficulties: Overview*. www.bdadyslexia.org.uk/dyslexic/dyslexia-and-specific-difficulties-overview.

British Psychological Society (2017) *Working with Interpreters: Guidelines for Psychologists*. www.bps.org.uk/news-and-policy/working-interpreters-guidelines-psychologists.

COI Communications (2001) *The Inquiry into the Management of the Care of Children Receiving Complex Heart Surgery at the Bristol Royal Infirmary*. http://webarchive.nationalarchives.gov.uk/+/http://www.dh.gov.uk/en/Publicationsandstatistics/Publications/PublicationsPolicyAndGuidance/DH_4005620.

Coyne, I.T. (1994) Parental participation in care: a critical review of the literature. *Journal of Advanced Nursing*, 21(4), 716–722.

Craft, M.J. and Craft, J.L. (1989) Perceived changes in siblings of hospitalized children: a comparison of sibling and parent reports. *Child Health Care*, 18(1), 42–48.

Croghan, E., Johnson, C. and Aveyard, P. (2004) School nurses: policies, working practices, roles and value perceptions. *Journal of Advanced Nursing*, 47(4), 377–385.

Darbyshire, P. (1994) *Living with a Sick Child in Hospital: The Experience of Parents and Nurses*. London, Chapman and Hall.

DCSF/DH (2007) *Teenage Parents Next Steps: Guidance for Local Authorities and Primary Care Trusts*. London, Department for Children, Schools and Families/Department of Health.

DCSF/DH (2009) *Healthy Lives, Brighter Futures: The Strategy for Children and Young People's Health*. London, Department for Children, Schools and Families/Department of Health.

Department of Health (2001) *Seeking Consent: Working with Children*. London, Department of Health.

Department of Health (2003) *Getting the Right Start. National Service Framework for Children. Standard for Hospital Services*. London, Department of Health.

Department of Health (2004) *Best Practice Guidance for Doctors and Other Health Professionals on the Provision of Advice and Treatment to Young People Under 16, on Contraceptive, Sexual and Reproductive Health*. London, Department of Health.

Department of Health (2008) *Carers at the Heart of 21st-century Families and Communities. 'A Caring System on your Side. A Life of your Own.'* London, Department of Health.

Department of Health (2015) *Future in Mind*. https://assets.publishing.service.gov.uk/government/uploads/system/uploads/attachment_data/file/414024/Childrens_Mental_Health.pdf.

Department of Health (2017) *You're Welcome Pilot 2017: Refreshed Standards for Piloting. Quality Criteria for Making Health Services Young People Friendly*. www.youngpeopleshealth.org.uk/yourewelcome/wp-content/uploads/2017/02/YoureWelcome_RefreshedsStandards.pdf.

DeVito, J.A. (2009) *The Interpersonal Communication Book* (12th edn). London, Pearson Education.

DfES (2004) *Every Child Matters: Change for Children*. London, Department for Education and Skills.

DfES (2005) *Common Core of Skills and Knowledge for the Children's Workforce*. London, Department for Education and Skills.

DfES (2006) *Youth Matters: Next Steps. Something to Do, Somewhere to Go, Someone to Talk To*. https://dera.ioe.ac.uk/7254/17/ACFA64E_Redacted.pdf.

Dunn, J. (2004) *Children's Friendships: The Beginnings of Intimacy*. Oxford, Blackwell.

Elliott, B. (2009) Communicating with children, young people and families in healthcare contexts. In A. Dunhill, B. Elliott and A. Shaw (eds), *Effective Communication and Engagement with Children and Young People, their Families and Carers* (pp. 73–87). Exeter, Learning Matters.

Gillick v West Norfolk and Wisbech AHA (1985) *AC112*. www.hrcr.org/safrica/childrens_rights/Gillick_WestNorfolk.htm.

Hargie, O. and Dickson, D. (2004) *Skilled Interpersonal Communication: Research, Theory and Practice* (4th edn). London, Routledge.

Hinduja, S. and Patchin, J.W. (2010) Bullying, cyberbulling and suicide. *Archives of Suicide Research*, 14(3), 206–221.

Hugman, B. (2009) *Healthcare Communication*. London, Pharmaceutical Press.

Hummelinck, A. and Pollock, K. (2006) Parents' information needs about the treatment of their chronically ill child: a qualitative study. *Patient Education and Counseling*, 62(2), 228–234.

Kelsey, J. and Abelson-Mitchell, N. (2007) Adolescent communication: perceptions and beliefs. *Journal of Children's and Young People's Nursing*, 1(1), 42–49.

Layard, R. and Hagell, A. (2015) *Healthy Young Minds: Transforming the Mental Health of Children*. World Innovation Summit for Health, Qatar, Qatar Foundation.

Leishman, J. (2004) Childhood and teenage pregnancies. *Nursing Standard*, 18(33), 33–36.

Lloyd, M. and Bor, R. (2004) *Communication Skills for Medicine* (2nd edn). Edinburgh, Churchill Livingstone.

Machin, K. and Watson, E. (2018) Recovery orientated practice. In K. Wright and M. McKeown (eds), *Essentials of Mental Health Nursing* (pp. 265–280). London, SAGE Publications.

Mathisen, L. and Butterworth, D. (2001) The role of play in hospitalisation of young children. *Neonatal, Pediatric and Child Health Nursing*, 4(3), 23–26.

Moss, B. (2008) *Communication Skills for Health and Social Care*. London, SAGE Publications.

National Association of Health Play Specialists (2018) *Guidelines for Professional Practice*. www.nahps.org.uk/publications/.

NHS Estates (2003) *Improving the Patient Experience: Friendly Healthcare Environments for Children and Young People*. London, HMSO.

NMC (2018) *The Code: Professional Standards of Practice and Behaviour for Nurses, Midwives and Nursing Associates*. www.nmc.org.uk/standards/code/.

NSPCC (2018) *Gillick Competency and Fraser Guidelines: Balancing Children's Rights with the Responsibility to Keep Them Safe from Harm*. https://learning.nspcc.org.uk/media/1541/gillick-competency-factsheet.pdf.

Ofcom (2017) *Children and Parents: Media Use and Attitudes Report*. www.ofcom.org.uk/__data/assets/pdf_file/0020/108182/children-parents-media-use-attitudes-2017.pdf.

O'Shea, E., Shea, J., Robert, T. and Cavanaugh, C. (2012) The needs of siblings of children with cancer: a nursing perspective. *Journal of Pediatric Oncology Nursing*, 29(4), 221–231.

PHE (2015) *A Framework for Supporting Teenage Mothers and Young Fathers*. http://dera.ioe.ac.uk/26423/1/PHE_LGA_Framework_for_supporting_teenage_mothers_and_young_fathers.pdf.

RCN (2009) *Mental Health in Children and Young People: A Toolkit for Nurses Who Are Not Mental Health Specialists*. London, Royal College of Nursing.

RCN (2013) *Adolescence: Boundaries and Connections. An RCN Guide for Working with Young People*. London, Royal College of Nursing.

RCN (2014) *Use of Digital Technology: Guidance for Nursing Staff Working with Children and Young People*. London, Royal College of Nursing.

Royal Society for Public Health (2017) *#Status of Mind: Social Media and Young People's Mental Health and Wellbeing*. www.rsph.org.uk/uploads/assets/uploaded/62be270a-a55f-4719-ad668c2ec7a74c2a.pdf.

Runeson, I. (2002) Children's participation in the decision-making process during hospitalization: an observational study. *Nursing Ethics*, 9(6), 583–598.

Sepion, B. (2009) Communicating with children and young people. In L. Childs, L. Coles and B. Marjoram (eds), *Essential Skills Clusters for Nurses: Theory for Practice* (pp. 19–28). Chichester, Wiley.

Shaw, A. (2009) Engaging with children, young people, families and carers at home and in other settings. In A. Dunhill, B. Elliott and A. Shaw (eds), *Effective Communication and Engagement with Children and Young People, their Families and Carers* (pp. 61–72). Exeter, Learning Matters.

Shields, L., Pratt, J. and Hunter, J. (2006) Family-centred care: a review of qualitative studies. *Journal of Clinical Nursing*, 15, 1317–1323.

Smith, L. and Callery, P. (2005) Children's accounts of their pre-operative information needs. *Journal of Clinical Nursing*, 14(2), 230–238.

Thompson, N. (2009) *People Skills* (3rd edn). Basingstoke, Palgrave Macmillan.

Young, B., Dixon-Woods, M., Windridge, K.C. and Heney, D. (2003) Managing communication with young people who have potentially life-threatening chronic illness: qualitative study of patients and parents. *British Medical Journal*, 326, 305.

FOURTEEN
COMMUNICATION AND THE COGNITIVELY IMPAIRED PATIENT

DUNCAN MITCHELL AND GARRY DIACK

.... THIS CHAPTER WILL HELP YOU TO

- Be proactive and creative in enhancing communication and understanding for people with cognitive impairment
- Assess and respond to carers and relatives in relation to information and consent
- Act collaboratively to enable and empower people to take a shared and active role in their care
- Make effective referrals to safeguard and protect children and vulnerable adults

Introduction

One of the recurring features of this book is that people are individuals and need to be treated as such. While this seems a rather obvious point, its failure in practice leads to many, if not most, communication problems. Sadly, there are many examples where a failure to communicate effectively has resulted in tragedy. An example can be found in the West Berkshire Safeguarding Adults Board (2016) *Safeguarding Adults Review*, in which it is reported that a patient died because her needs were not communicated between different care agencies.

This chapter examines the general approach that nurses need to take when nursing people with cognitive impairments. It will focus on the needs of service users who have some form of cognitive impairment that requires specific communication skills in response. It will explore the nature of mental impairment and offer some golden rules that nurses need when caring for people with cognitive impairments. It will use specific conditions as examples and introduce you to some guidance that will help you to adapt your skills to working with people with specific conditions.

Why does cognitive impairment present a communication problem for nurses?

Adults and children with some form of cognitive impairment are just as likely as anyone else to access a broad range of health services, particularly children with learning difficulties (Edbrooke-Childs et al., 2017). Patients may have a range of communication difficulties from having no speech at all to having difficulty understanding complex language or concepts. Some people may use a form of symbol communication such as British Sign Language (BSL) or Makaton. In much the same way as people have different levels of competence around verbal communication, so too may the person with a learning disability have a limited, and very personal, range of signing abilities. Some people will have a permanent impairment due to an acquired brain injury or dementia, or a developmental impairment such as autism or Down's syndrome. Some patients may have a temporary impairment due to an acute illness or toxic state, such as an infection and high temperature, or lack of oxygen, both of which can cause confusion. Confusion can affect both the person's ability to understand what someone else is saying and their ability to communicate their needs. People with serious mental illnesses may also have altered and fluctuating abilities to understand because the illness interferes with functional thinking, concentration and attention.

School nurses will have experience with children with learning disabilities, learning difficulties and autism spectrum disorders who often present with styles of communication which their families and education carers have adapted to but which present a barrier to health professionals. The very unique and personal forms of communication between family members and carers with a long history of involvement with a person will sometimes require interpretation. For example, a particular tilt of the head, raising of the eyebrow or certain vocalisation will be full of meaning for someone with knowledge of the person but may be missed by a professional who only has periodic engagement with that person. It can be useful in general care settings for nurses to strive to understand and adopt the communication styles used by family and carers because these are not only effective but are familiar to the patient and reduce anxiety and improve recovery (Callery and Milnes, 2012; Kornhaber et al., 2016; Price, 2017). In order to do this successfully it is important for the health professional to establish a strong working relationship with the family and carers to build a comprehensive understanding of the nuances of the person's communication. It is also very important to ensure that adequate time is allowed for the person to communicate (Hemsley et al., 2012). In many fields of care, nurses will encounter patients with acquired cognitive impairments such as dementia or stroke, whose communication abilities are likely to be limited by disorientation, poor short-term memory and emotional lability (being prone to strong and fluctuating emotions).

What are cognitive impairments?

To understand terms that seem complicated it is usually necessary to break them down into manageable sections. So, to help with understanding of the term cognitive impairment each word will be defined before looking at the term itself.

> *Cognitive*: the noun form of this word is cognition and this means 'the mental processes by which knowledge is acquired' (Oxford University Press, 2002:144). For example, it is cognitive skills that will determine the understanding of a message given to you by someone else.
>
> *Impairment*: this means a damaging or weakening of a function or process.

So, put together, the two words mean a compromised or weakened ability to understand information. It is important to understand that this is about knowledge, not about emotion. For example, you might have heard a phrase like 'just because I'm slow it doesn't mean that I don't have feelings.' See Practice example box 14.1 for a short patient example where the key points are separated in order to identify the cognitive impairment.

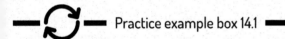 Practice example box 14.1

A young man with learning disabilities arrives in the emergency department

Mark, a young man with learning disabilities, arrives at the emergency department. He has been involved in a road traffic accident. He was hit by a car while walking on the pavement and has a badly damaged right leg (physical injury).

He is confused because he is in shock (natural response).

However, even when he isn't in shock, he finds it difficult to understand things quickly, especially when events are unexpected or unfamiliar. Mark cannot understand what has happened to him because he has always been told that it is safe to walk on the pavement where cars cannot hit you. Mark is also uncertain about what might take place in the hospital (cognitive impairment).

He is in a lot of pain from his leg injury and is very frightened and upset (natural response).

Later in this chapter we will come back to this example to see why it is so important to be able to understand that some people have cognitive impairments.

First, let's have a look at the range of the things that might involve cognitive impairment.

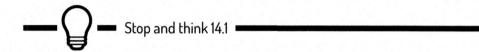

Stop and think 14.1

Make a list of the sort of things that you think might involve a cognitive impairment.

There are a range of conditions that might be included in your list. Some examples follow but they are by no means the only ones:

- Learning disability: sometimes also known as developmental disability or intellectual disability
- Dementia: usually but not always affecting older people
- Brain damage following an accident
- Brain damage following a stroke
- Some mental health conditions
- Drug/alcohol intoxication.

This list is a simple one and each condition can be split into different aspects. Some of the conditions are short term and others are longer term or permanent. This chapter is not designed to give you information about each condition. That would be a book in itself. For example, if we were to look just at learning disability the definition is far from fixed and covers a very wide range of people. At one extreme are people who need support with basic needs such as eating and drinking, toileting and dressing, and at the other extreme are people who have difficulty in their learning but require few if any specialist services. An estimate of the number of people in England with learning disabilities made in 2015 by the Learning Disability Observatory was 1,087,100. It is worth noting that only 23% of people with learning disabilities are identified on GP registers. This means that 77% of people, the 'hidden majority', are not identified in data collection exercises (Hatton et al., 2016).

Basic assessment of cognitive impairment

Nurses in all fields of practice are expected to be able to make assessments of patient need and this will include communication ability. Nurses are sometimes worried that this means that they are required to make specialist assessments of the wide range of conditions that they come across in their field of practice, however, that is not the case. Nurses need to be able to identify whether someone has an understanding of what is being communicated to them. This usually means using a process called positive clarification in order to check for understanding. For example, asking the person to repeat back what they have heard in their own words. If there is a problem, then nurses need to be able to examine and adapt their own communication method. This may mean speaking more slowly, altering their voice tonality (**voice prosody**), using less complex sentences and allowing more time for a response (remember the models in Chapter 1, showing that communication works at least two directions). Nurses then need to know when to refer for specialist help and where to make that referral to. See Box 14.1 for a case study example from the Department of Constitutional Affairs' Mental Capacity Act 2005 Code of Practice.

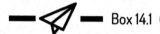 Box 14.1

Example of capacity issues from Code of Practice of the Mental Capacity Act

Mr Elliott is 87 years old and lives alone. He has poor short-term memory, and he often forgets to eat. He also sometimes neglects his personal hygiene. His daughter talks to him about moving into residential care. She decides that he understands the reasons for her concerns as well as the risks of continuing to live alone and, having weighed these up, he has the capacity to decide to stay at home and accept the consequences.

Two months later, Mr Elliott has a fall and breaks his leg. While being treated in hospital, he becomes confused and depressed. He says he wants to go home, but the staff think that the deterioration in his mental health has affected his capacity to make this decision at this time. They think he cannot understand the consequences or weigh up the risks he faces if he goes home. They refer him to a specialist in old age psychiatry who assesses whether his mental health is affecting his capacity to make this decision. The staff will then use the specialist's opinion to help their assessment of Mr Elliott's capacity.

(Department of Constitutional Affairs, 2007:57)

In this example staff believe that there may be an issue about Mr Elliott's cognitive ability and his capacity to make a decision. The Mental Capacity Act (2005) is very clear that professionals have to assume that people have capacity to make decisions unless they have reasons not to. It is the communication skills of nurses that will help them to decide whether people have the capacity to make decisions, and have the ability to communicate their wishes.

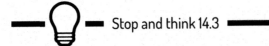

Stop and think 14.2

In the case study above, consider what might give you cause to think that Mr Elliott's mental health is deteriorating. What sort of ways could you use to communicate with Mr Elliott to help with your assessment?

It is most likely that staff have noticed that Mr Elliott's memory has deteriorated. This might be his short-term or his long-term memory, or possibly both. The signs may have been that Mr Elliott was slow to recognise someone he knew, forgets that he has eaten a meal or does not always know where he is. He may be struggling to find the correct words for common objects, or perhaps gets his words mixed up.

To help assess Mr Elliott, the staff will have to spend time with him and try to look at everything he is saying rather than isolate some elements that might seem confusing. Any perceived pressure might lead Mr Elliott to feel that he is being tested by the staff. It is important to speak clearly and listen carefully to all aspects of his communication. This will include taking note of the speed of his responses, his body language, where and who he looks at when answering and whether or not he looks anxious or upset. It is also important not to ask the same question in lots of different ways. Remember that your assessment at this point is to find out whether there is a need to ask for a specialist assessment.

When talking to people, remember that some questions seem very strange and it is not always easy to remember simple things. If someone asked you what you had for your meal last night, would you remember?

It is common for nurses to have to make quick assessments when they first meet people. While patients may have notes that list underlying conditions, this may not always be the case. Some nurses may say that they have insufficient information about cognitive impairments and have to make decisions about the help that people might need.

Stop and think 14.3

See the case study in Box 14.2 below. What sort of things would you ask a person in order to find out if they have a learning disability?

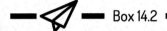 **Box 14.2**

The knowledge of healthcare staff

A staff nurse who is fairly new to a medical assessment ward assesses a newly admitted young woman who has intermittent severe abdominal pain. The woman has come to hospital by ambulance but is otherwise on her own. The nurse suspects that the woman has learning disabilities because she answers her questions very slowly and doesn't seem to understand what is happening to her. The hospital has a care pathway for people with learning disabilities but the nurse is not sure whether the woman has been diagnosed with a learning disability and she doesn't know how to broach the subject.

There is no absolute list for this sort of informal assessment but, in order to know whether someone has a learning disability, the following questions (Box 14.3) will help.

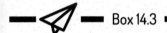 **Box 14.3**

RCN guidance on learning disabilities for nursing staff

- Ask the person if they have learning disabilities.
- Does the person have a social worker, care manager or key worker?
- Did the person go to a special school or attend mainstream school with special support?
- Does the person go to a day centre?
- Has the person ever been seen by learning disability staff or lived in a learning disability hospital?
- Can the person read or write?
- Can the person tell the time?
- Does the person have difficulty in communicating?
- Can the person remember certain everyday facts about themselves (where they live, their birthday)?

(RCN, 2006:3)

Of course, you would not be expected to ask questions according to the whole list. Some of the questions would be part of a standard assessment (such as date of birth). Some of the questions would be very difficult to answer for the woman when she is in pain. However, they would help you to understand whether someone is cognitively impaired due to learning disability.

The nurses' role in assessment is therefore important in helping to understand whether people are cognitively impaired and whether specific communication techniques are needed. It is important to remember that an impairment does not define everything about an individual, nor, as will be seen in the next section, does it provide a model for communication.

Communication with people with cognitive impairments

There are some golden rules in communication with people with cognitive impairments:

- Always address the patient first and if you need to speak to a relative or carer then you must ensure that you keep returning to the patient as the main focus of your interaction.
- Be aware that the person's carer may be used to offering interpretations and opinions on behalf of the person.
- Never assume that someone does not understand what you are saying. They will be used to people trying to communicate with them and they will have learned at least some aspects of the communication process.
- Remember that it takes at least two people to communicate – it may be the way you are giving the message that stops someone understanding.
- Remember to allow sufficient time for the communication to take place.
- Make sure that you have the person's attention: a person with a learning disability may have quite a short concentration span. Pace your questions accordingly.
- Never blame the patient for not understanding. Ask yourself if there is another way to put your point/question across – showing your impatience could also add to the problem.
- Always find out if the person uses any communication aids.
- Always use very clear and concrete language and avoid colloquial or ambiguous terms such as 'under the weather'.
- Remember that many people want to please others and will give answers even if they don't understand the question. This may be made more complicated if you nod your head when asking a question. (Try this with a partner or friend: ask them if they want a cup of tea while nodding your head. Then ask them if they felt any subtle pressure to accept a cup, even though they may not have wanted one.)
- Always treat people with respect.

These rules are not exclusive and you may want to add your own points to the list. You will certainly need to add other communication approaches learned from this book. You may think that some are common sense; they should be, but if they were always practised then people would not need to be constantly reminded about them. You might also think that some or all of them apply to all patients, not just those who are cognitively impaired. In this you would be quite right.

There is one further golden rule that requires a little more explanation. The rule is to avoid assuming that a physical symptom is part of someone's cognitive impairment. This is sometimes known as **diagnostic overshadowing**. The *RCN Bulletin* poses the question:

> If someone with a learning disability is admitted to hospital banging their head, being silent or laughing, do you assume that's part of their behaviour? Or might it signal they are in pain or distress?
>
> (RCN, 2018:1)

The RCN suggests that diagnostic overshadowing leads to poorer healthcare for people with mental illness or learning disability, contributing to the lower life expectancy of this population group. However, many people with learning disabilities are supported by other people – such as family members or care staff – and this may help the nurse interpret the behaviour. It is sometimes really important to involve such people in care and this often helps avoid diagnostic overshadowing. An influential research report by Mencap found that:

> Parents and family members can often provide vital information that can help doctors and nurses to decide on appropriate treatments for people with a learning disability. But there appears to be a tendency among healthcare professionals to discount this information, or not even to consult family members in the first place. It is often assumed that they are over-emotional, irrational and uninformed. By disregarding the views and information that family members provide, doctors can make diagnoses, leading to premature, avoidable deaths.
>
> (Mencap, 2007:19)

There is sometimes a tension between both protecting confidentiality and keeping the person at the heart of decision-making and involving family members and other carers. Some people may not want their families involved in some aspects of their care and it is always important to have informed consent. However, many people would see their involvement as natural and it is often families and carers who know most about the people they care for.

Consent

One issue that often confuses nurses is whether they can give treatment to a patient who cannot give clear consent. Sometimes this is when a patient cannot give written consent, and sometimes when they appear to withhold consent by their actions (such as shying away from having an injection). This is usually an issue of communication and involves sensitive talking and listening.

Box 14.4 gives another example from the Mental Health Act Code of Practice.

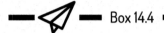 **Box 14.4**

Consent issues

Luke, a young man, was seriously injured in a road traffic accident and suffered permanent brain damage. He has been in hospital several months, and has made good progress, but he gets very frustrated at his inability to concentrate or do things for himself.

Luke now needs surgical treatment on his leg. During the early morning ward round, the surgeon tries to explain what is involved in the operation. She asks Luke to sign a consent form, but he gets angry and says he doesn't want to talk about it.

His key nurse knows that Luke becomes more alert and capable later in the day. After lunch she asks him if he would like to discuss the operation again. She also knows that he responds better one to one than in a group. So, she takes Luke into a private room and repeats the information that the surgeon gave him earlier. He understands why the treatment is needed, what is involved and the likely consequences. Therefore, Luke has the capacity to make a decision about the operation.

(Department of Constitutional Affairs, 2007:37)

The Code of Practice for the Mental Capacity Act (2005) (Department of Constitutional Affairs, 2007) is concerned with much more than capacity for consent to treatment, but it helps provide the framework that nurses need when communicating with people with cognitive impairments. In the example above the nurse knows that it takes time to help her patient to understand a procedure and to consent to it.

Priorities for care

Now we are going to return to the first short case study of this chapter. Look again at the example of Mark in Practice example box 14.1.

Some of the care that Mark needs will be exactly the same as anyone else with a similar injury. His injury will need to be assessed and a decision made about whether treatment is urgent.

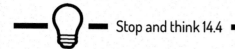 Stop and think 14.4

Think about how Mark's cognitive impairment might affect his response to initial assessment and treatment. What are the ways in which you would communicate with Mark?

Mark's cognitive impairment means that he may not see the connection between his accident and being in hospital. He may confuse being in hospital with other times that he has had treatment. It is likely that he will take a long time to understand information, and the pain that he is experiencing will make this even more difficult for him.

It is important to remember the golden rules. Speak to Mark directly: he will understand some of what you are saying and you can ask him questions to check his understanding. Mark may have limited speech but you can use touch to communicate especially if trying to locate areas of pain and, if it is possible, find out if Mark uses any communication aids. Give Mark plenty of time to absorb information and don't give him lots of information or ask lots of different questions at once. Do many of the things that you would do with any other patient, in particular being reassuring and calm. There will need to be an assessment of Mark's mental capacity to consent to treatment and if Mark is unable to consent then the team will need to consider a 'best interests' decision.

For further reading see the Mental Capacity Act Code of Practice (Department of Constitutional Affairs, 2007).

While Mark's cognitive impairment is unlikely to change, the shock will diminish, as will his being frightened and upset. It is therefore important that assessment of understanding continues during and after treatment.

Communication techniques for people with severe cognitive impairment

Sometimes we may have a patient who is unable to speak or who is unable to comprehend their environment or the people around them. This may be due to an altered state of consciousness such as a comatose patient, someone in an acute or chronic confusional state due to poor memory retention or impaired concentration, or someone who is very distracted by impaired thought processes. As mentioned earlier in this chapter, many people with communication difficulties may rely on communication aids. The RCN Northern Ireland (2018) identify some of the aids that can be used by general and learning disability nurses and specialist practitioners:

- Personal Communication Passports
- easy-to-read formats (i.e. information leaflets and posters)
- Makaton
- signing (BSL)
- picture cards
- Talking Mats.

These can be physical aids such as picture cards or techniques such as Makaton, a simple sign language commonly used in the UK that uses gestures or pictures for simplified communication. Personal Communication Passports can be actual booklets or be in digital format, and help facilitate information-giving to health professionals. As they are about the individual person, they help staff understand the person's care needs, but also likes and dislikes, ensuring more individualised care (Hammond, 2018). Talking Mats are a commercially produced tool that can be used with children or people with communication difficulties (Scottish Health Council, 2019).

More complex techniques such as Augmentative and Alternative Communication (AAC) may be used in specialist education and care areas (Enderby et al., 2013), and it may be worth finding out about an individual patient's needs and abilities from their usual carers regarding common and useful techniques that can be used that the person will understand.

Look at the links in the Further reading section at the end of this chapter for more information on the communication aids.

People with specific cognitive impairments are likely to have functional strengths that can be used for communication and understanding. Older dementia patients, for example, often have varied levels of impairments in different cognitive areas. Hall (1988) identified four different areas of impairment common in dementia patients:

1   intellectual loss: memory, attention, sense of time
2   affective/personality loss: raised anxiety, emotional blunting
3   planning loss: loss of functional thinking – can't plan or problem-solve
4   low stress threshold: inability to tolerate stress, frustration leading to emotional lability (easily provoked to anger, crying, laughing).

These different areas of impairment mean that the person may have strengths in one but not another. So, a patient with an impaired memory may still understand on an emotional level and so recognise kindness – or anger – and learn to trust or distrust a person, even when they don't know who that person is.

Rantz and McShane (1995) made a study of nursing home staff who worked with chronically confused patients and found four nursing interventions that improved communication and understanding and so reduced patient anxiety and distress:

1 interpreting reality: use of familiar objects in the patient's environment such as photos or mementos
2 maintaining normality: having a routine that can be understood by the patients on a behavioural level
3 meeting basic needs: for exercise, reducing boredom and social activities
4 monitoring for signs of distress: good observation skills, using the individual patient's ways of communicating distress such as agitation, crying, withdrawal, reluctance or changes in behaviour.

Sometimes, simply being with someone, holding their hand or just spending time with them can communicate an idea of trust and togetherness. Even a person who does not know who the nurse is will gain an emotional relationship with them. This is referred to as **transference** and describes a situation where one person relates emotionally to another as if they were someone else, and a previous relationship appears to be re-enacted in the nurse–patient relationship (Brim, 2014). See Box 14.5 for an example.

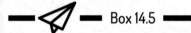 **Box 14.5**

Transference for a patient with cognitive impairment

Mr G was an older man with moderate memory loss. He could not remember day-to-day events and frequently confused nurses for members of his family. Mr G's key nurse developed a trusting relationship with him and became one of the few people Mr G would trust to be near him when he got confused and distressed. He could never remember the nurse's name but often called her by his daughter's name.

In this example, Mr G appears to have used emotional memory to understand his relationship with his key nurse. He has unconsciously transferred his memories of his daughter to someone who 'reminds him' of his daughter on an emotional level. This kind of relating is common in many intense counselling and psychotherapy relationships but also occurs quite easily with people whose intellectual abilities are impaired or suppressed and therefore who do not present a rationalising barrier to what is a purely emotional level of relating (Bateman and Holmes, 1995).

Conclusion

This chapter has introduced you to communication with people who have cognitive impairments. You now know about different cognitive impairments and some of the ways in which they affect communication. You now also know some golden rules about nursing people with cognitive impairments. The key to working with people with cognitive impairments is to treat them individually and with respect. You can add lessons from this chapter to those that you have learned from the rest of this book.

FURTHER READING

Communication Matters (nd) *What is AAC?* www.communicationmatters.org.uk/page/what-is-aac.
Personal Communication Passports. www.communicationpassports.org.uk/Home/.
Makaton. www.makaton.org/.
RCN (2017) *The Needs of People with Learning Disabilities: What Pre-Registration Students Should Know*. London, Royal College of Nursing.
Talking Mats. www.talkingmats.com/talking-mats-interview-tool/.

REFERENCES

Bateman, A. and Holmes, J. (1995) *Introduction to Psychoanalysis: Contemporary Theory and Practice*. Hove, Brunner-Routledge.
Brim, V. (2014) Using the concepts of transference and counter-transference in care management supervision. *Journal of Aging Life Care*, Fall 2014. www.aginglifecarejournal.org/using-the-concepts-of-transference-and-counter-transference-in-care-management-supervision/.
Callery, P. and Milnes, L. (2012) Communication between nurses, children and their parents in asthma review consultations. *Journal of Clinical Nursing*, 21(11–12), 1641–1650.
Department of Constitutional Affairs (2007) *Mental Capacity Act Code of Practice*. London, DCA. https://webarchive.nationalarchives.gov.uk/+/http://www.dca.gov.uk/legal-policy/mental-capacity/mca-cp.pdf
Edbrooke-Childs, J., Deighton, J. and Wolpert, M. (2017) Changes in severity of psychosocial difficulties in adolescents accessing specialist mental healthcare in England (2009–2014). *Journal of Adolescence*, 60, 47–52.
Enderby, P., Judge, S., Creer, S. and John, A.U. (2013) *Communication Matters – Research Matters: An AAC Evidence Base Beyond the Anecdote Examining the Need for, and Provision of, AAC in the United Kingdom*. Sheffield, University of Sheffield/Barnsley Hospital.
Hall, G. (1988) Care of the patient with Alzheimer's disease at home. *Nursing Clinics of North America*, 23, 31–46.
Hammond, R. (2018) Communication Passports: giving a voice to those with learning disabilities. *Nursing Times*. www.nursingtimes.net/students/communication-passports-giving-a-voice-to-those-with-learning-disabilities/7023130.article.
Hatton, C., Glover, G., Emerson, E. and Brown, I. (2016) *People with Learning Disabilities in England 2015: Main Report*. London, Public Health England.
Hemsley, B., Balandin, S. and Worrall, L. (2012) Nursing the patient with complex communication needs: time as a barrier and a facilitator to successful communication in hospital. *Journal of Advanced Nursing*, 68(1), 116–126.
Kornhaber, R., Walsh, K., Duff, J. and Walker, K. (2016) Enhancing adult therapeutic interpersonal relationships in the acute health care setting: an integrative review. *Journal of Multidisciplinary Healthcare*, 9, 537–546.

Mencap (2007) *Death by Indifference*. London, Mencap.

Oxford University Press (2002) *Oxford Concise Medical Dictionary* (6th edn). Oxford, Oxford University Press.

Price, B. (2017) Managing patients' anxiety about planned medical interventions. *Nursing Standard*, 31(47), 53–61.

Rantz, M. and McShane, R. (1995) Nursing interventions for chronically confused home residents. *Geriatric Nursing*, 16, 22–27.

RCN (2006) *Meeting the Health Needs of People with Learning Disabilities: Guidance for Nursing Staff*. London, Royal College of Nursing.

RCN (2018) All you see isn't all there is; looking beyond learning disability to recognise the physical symptoms of ill health. *RCN Bulletin*, 15 May.

RCN Northern Ireland (2018) *The Registered Nurse – Learning Disability: Skills, Knowledge and Expertise across the Lifespan*. London, Royal College of Nursing.

Scottish Health Council (2019) *Talking Mats*. http://scottishhealthcouncil.org/patient_public_participation/participation_toolkit/talking_mats.aspx#.XLxzzOhKgb4.

West Berkshire Safeguarding Adults Board (2016) *Report of Learning Together Safeguarding Adults Review into the Case of Mrs H*. www.sabberkshirewest.co.uk/media/1279/mrs-h-report-july-2016-final-report-published-8-june-2017.pdf.

FIFTEEN
ENGAGEMENT, MOTIVATION AND CHANGING BEHAVIOUR
MAXINE HOLT AND CLEMENTINAH ROOKE

.... THIS CHAPTER WILL HELP YOU TO:

- Help people use their strengths to achieve their goals and aspirations
- Empower and support patient choice
- Promote health and wellbeing, self-care and independence
- Address sensitive issues for individuals, communities and populations
- Work within a public health framework to assess and plan care

Introduction

This chapter builds on the health promotion strategies addressed in Chapter 9. It considers how the theories of the Health Belief Model and the Behaviour Change Model support nurses in delivering health promotion and behaviour change in practice settings.

When we deliver health promotion interventions, one important assessment feature is identifying and understanding the attitudes, beliefs and values our patients have regarding their health and wellbeing. Ideally, exploration of these variables should be done with the patient or groups we are working with. Once they are identified we can tailor interventions to help motivate our patients to adopt healthier lifestyles. First, let's consider the theories behind health beliefs.

The Health Belief Model

This is an established model of health beliefs from Rosenstock (1974). The theory underpinning the Health Belief Model (sometimes called the HBM) is that the perceived threat of disease serves as a motivator for the patient to take action. Health promotion therefore is about communicating to patients that behaviours like smoking or poor diet may lead to coronary heart disease and stroke. This information can be used to motivate the patient to change behaviour and reduce their risk of disease (Figure 15.1).

The Health Belief Model can be an effective framework with which nurses can evaluate patients' health behaviour and deliver interventions. Nurses have used this model effectively for health promotion for breast cancer screening (Medina-Shepherd and Kleier, 2010), smoking cessation (Schofield et al., 2007), mapping and improving sexual health behaviour (Browes, 2006) and treatment choice for obesity (Armstrong et al., 2009). Recent evidence also supports the use of the Health Belief Model for application to type 2 diabetes mellitus (Noushirvani and Mansouri, 2018), leisure noise/hearing health in young people (Gilliver et al., 2015), anxiety disorders (Langley et al., 2018) and prevention services (Luquis and Kensinger, 2019).

We can explore the elements of the model that are outlined in Figure 15.1.

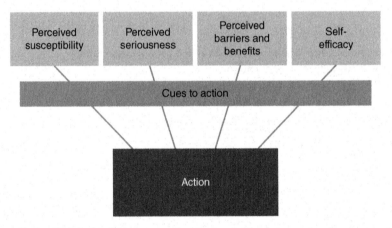

Figure 15.1 The Health Belief Model

Perceived susceptibility (am I going to get the disease?)

Most of the time people tend to think that they are less likely to develop a health problem compared to other people. Therefore, some people don't think health information is relevant to them. An example of this is health promotion campaigns on the increasing risks of HIV transmission among heterosexuals.

Here's an example of a nurse–patient conversation:

Nurse: 'Jenny, you mentioned you don't have a steady partner at the moment so I'd advise you that it's better to use condoms as well as the pill, to protect yourself against sexually transmitted diseases, including HIV.'

Patient: 'Oh, I don't need to worry about HIV. I'm not the type to be at risk.'

Perceived seriousness (how bad would it be?)

Some patients believe that it is better to leave things alone at the moment and perhaps return to thinking about it in the future.

Nurse: 'Sam, your blood pressure is a little on the high side. We need to think how we might help to reduce it. I wonder if you might consider losing some weight? Losing even 10% of your weight will help lower your blood pressure. What do you think?'

Patient: 'I'll give it some thought maybe but perhaps later when I get back from my holiday, or after Christmas maybe. Besides, my dad was fat and lived to a ripe old age and his mother was thin and she died in her 50s. Anyway nurse, when your time's up that's it. You've got to go sometime.'

Perceived barriers and benefits (will it be easy to get something done about it? What will it cost me?)

Here the person weighs the pros and cons. It is based on the fact that the person must believe that a change in behaviour will benefit them. These costs are weighed up not just in financial terms but against other areas of their lives.

Nurse: 'Reducing your lithium medication when you're so stressed is putting you at risk of becoming manic.'

Patient: 'I know, but the stress is down to the amount of work I have to get through right now, and being just a bit high helps me get through it quickly.'

Self-efficacy (is it possible for me to do something about it? What are the things that might stop me?)

Patients will consider whether the time is right for them and think about the possible negative outcomes.

Nurse: 'Mary, we have discussed the fact that if you carry on smoking 30 a day you are at risk from developing smoking-related diseases. Could you consider how you might stop smoking using one of the therapies we have discussed?'

Patient: 'I'm not sure I can do it. I know, you see, the minute I give up I will put loads of weight on and I don't want that.'

Cues to action – take action (OK, I am ready to make a change)

The model proposes that some patients need cues to change some health-related behaviour, such as a change in their appearance, a death of a close family member or a comment from a close friend, relative or significant other. As nurses, we can sometimes be the significant other. Once this happens, the patient is ready to make a change based on having the correct information and an improved motivation to change. See the case study in Box 15.1.

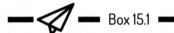 Box 15.1

Giving information to facilitate change

Alan is staff nurse on a paediatric ward caring for Jimmy who is seriously ill with measles. Jimmy's mother visits every day after dropping her other two children off at the nursery. She tells Alan that none of her children have been immunised against measles as she doesn't believe in immunisations anyway. After getting to know her, Alan asks about her concerns regarding vaccination, and he is able to allay some of her fears. He asks whether she would now consider having her other two children immunised to protect them from the effects the disease has had on Jimmy. She agrees and he arranges an appointment for her in the local clinic.

We have a responsibility to communicate the need for our patients to consider healthier lifestyles to prevent disease. Understanding our patients' beliefs about their health and wellbeing is an important factor in communicating health promotion. It enables the patient to feel valued and listened to. The Health Belief Model cannot predict behaviour or identify which factors are important in influencing behaviour change. However, it does enable us to consider overall the complex range of factors that influence a person's health behaviour.

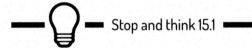 Stop and think 15.1

Think back over your placement experiences so far and about some of the patients you have recently cared for. In conversations about their health needs, can you use the main aspects of the Health Belief Model to identify the range of factors which may have influenced their health behaviour?

- Perceived susceptibility (am I going to get the disease?)
- Perceived seriousness (how bad would it be?)
- Perceived barriers and benefits (will it be easy to get something done about it? What will it cost me?)
- Self-efficacy (Is it possible for me to do something about it? What are the things that might stop me?)
- Cues to action – take action (OK, I am ready to make a change)

If you were to meet these patients on placement again, how might you respond differently in conversations you had?

There are some inherent limitations associated with the Health Belief Model. For example, it could be argued that it assumes that health behaviour is rational and that it appears to place too much emphasis on the individual ignoring the social and economic context. It is, therefore, important that we exercise great caution and avoid blind application of the theory (Coulson et al., 2016).

The Behaviour Change Model

Another useful model is offered by Prochaska and DiClemente (1986). The Behaviour Change Model considers how patients make health-related behavioural decisions, the stages they go through and how they move from one stage to another. The model focuses on *how* people change rather than *why*. The model is based on sequential stages:

- pre-contemplation
- contemplation
- preparation to change
- action for change
- maintenance
- relapse.

The model is characterised very much like a revolving door, and the length of time spent in each stage varies. Throughout each stage people are occupied by different physical and mental processes (Figure 15.2).

Pre-contemplation

A patient in the pre-contemplative stage does not intend to make any change to their health behaviour in the foreseeable future. Patients may be in this stage because they are uninformed

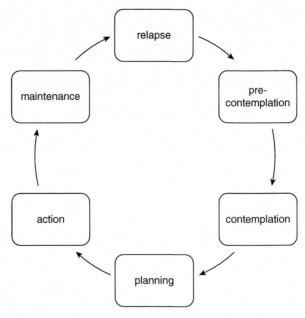

Figure 15.2 The Behaviour Change Model

or not really interested about the consequences of their behaviour, or they may have tried to change in the past and been unsuccessful.

> Patient: 'Sorry nurse but, before you start about my smoking, I've tried everything and nothing works for me so I just have to face it I will always be a smoker. Anyway, my dad was a smoker and lived to a good age.'

Contemplation

Patients here are thinking about their health and lifestyle behaviour and intending to do something about it, usually in a given time scale, and can often stay in this stage for a very long time or may never actually move forward at all.

> Patient: 'I know I am probably drinking too much but my job makes it hard to change. I'd like to do something about it but don't know what.'

Preparation to change

This is the stage in which the patient is intending to take action in the immediate future. Again, this may be measured in time, for example in the next month. Some patients we work with may already have made a move to taking action, such as joining a gym.

Patient: 'I have thought about getting more exercise but I'm too embarrassed to go to a gym. Someone suggested getting a dog. Do you think that actually works?'

Action for change

This is the stage in which patients have made specific obvious changes in their health behaviours and lifestyles in the past 6 months. This stage involves clear and realistic time-planned goals which are supported by others to ensure success.

Patient: 'I feel so much better. I've lost 6 kilograms in weight and my breathing has improved. I seem to have plateaued out though. Should I increase my exercise or reduce my calorie intake?'

Maintenance

Patients in the maintenance stage are working to prevent relapse and a return to their old health and lifestyle behaviours. The new health behaviour therefore becomes a normal pattern. Many patients find this a difficult stage and many people relapse and revert back to any of the above stages.

Patient: 'It's been a year now since I felt really depressed. People say I have changed – that I'm more outgoing. It's difficult, sometimes, to not give in to the negative thoughts, but I try to remember the CBT steps and I think the switching to positive thinking is becoming a habit.'

Relapse

A patient may relapse to an earlier stage. It is important that we provide positive support and not allow the patient to consider themselves as having failed, but are encouraged to review their action plans and recognise that relapse is a part of the process of change.

Patient: 'Oh I feel so annoyed with myself! I was doing so well and then I went to a party and ate loads. I've been binging ever since. I am back to square one now: it's hopeless.'

Prochaska et al. (1994) modified the model and added a further stage described as 'termination or final stage' in which people experience no temptation to return to their old behaviour patterns.

Despite its wide use and popularity, to date the Behaviour Change Model has also attracted substantial scholarly criticism targeting the 'stages of change' construct within the model (Coulson et al., 2016). Unfortunately, these debates are beyond the scope of this chapter. However, it would be prudent that we consider these in our efforts to help the behaviour of those whom we care for.

The models in action

Let's consider how both of the above models can be applied to our work in communicating with patients about health issues. It is useful to have a guide on how to get started and Ewles and Simnett (Scriven, 2017) and Rollnick et al. (2007) provide us with some tips on how to do this (Figure 15.3).

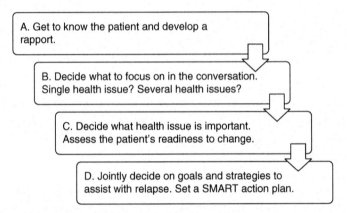

Figure 15.3 Model of how to engage patients in behaviour change. The SMART action plan is discussed later in this chapter
Source: adapted from Ewles and Simnett (Scriven, 2017) and Rollnick et al. (2007)

Using the previous case scenarios, we'll consider each of these steps in working with a patient from the pre-contemplation stage through the whole cycle and how we communicate with patients to effect change.

Get to know the patient and develop a rapport

Nursing is a very busy job but it is important that we do not skip or ignore this stage as it is in the early interactions that the nurse–patient relationship is formed. This stage is when the patient gains the first impression of us and how interested we are in them as individuals. Firstly, we need to ensure we are in an appropriate environment. A patient's bedside on a noisy ward or a busy waiting room is not the best place to initiate a discussion with a patient. A private interview room with interesting materials which communicate health issues, such as posters, leaflets and reading materials, is a good place to start. We need to get to know the patient, what their beliefs and knowledge about their health and wellbeing are and whether they are ready to change. One useful way in getting to know the patient is by using narratives or stories, for example getting the patient to talk about what a typical day is like for them.

When using this approach, the nurse asks the patient to take them through a journey of their typical day in relation to a health behaviour or health problem. In other words, the patient is painting a picture that we can use to better understand them. The following is a case scenario about a patient in the pre-contemplation stage called John, whose heavy smoking is contributing to his chest problems and breathlessness.

Nurse: 'John, how can I help you with the problem you're having with your chest?'

Patient: 'Sorry nurse but before you start about my smoking, I've tried everything and nothing really works for me so I just have to face it, I will always be a smoker. Anyway, my dad was a smoker and lived to a good age.'

Nurse: 'OK, I understand, but perhaps we'll just begin by getting to know each other a little. Maybe you could tell me what a typical day is like for you with your chest, from when you get up in the morning. Is that OK?'

The skill we need to apply here is one of listening and only interrupting if really necessary and with very simple questions. Rollnick et al. (2007) suggest that you will know that you have got the balance right if you are only doing 10–15% of the talking.

Decide what to focus on in the conversation

Some patients will have a number of health behaviours that they want to discuss and this can make it difficult for both the nurse and the patient to know where to start.

Nurse: 'John, it seems that there are a number of things you are concerned about. These are your chest, weight and that you cannot get out and exercise. Perhaps we can look at which ones are most important to you and begin there? How about we list which issues cause you problems in your day-to-day life and you put them in order of importance?'

The nurse should not rush into the discussion but ascertain what is (or are) the most important issues that the patient can focus on at that time. It is important to note that a patient may only be able to focus on one behaviour change at a time. Also, it is worth remembering that a change in one health behaviour may have a positive effect on another, which can act as a powerful motivator.

Nurse: 'I know you've had a poor experience with nicotine gum and it's put you off thinking about giving up smoking. How about we look at this again and see what else might help you in giving up smoking. If we can improve your chest it will help you to get out and about and exercise more, which will help with your weight loss. How does that sound?'

Is the patient ready to change?

Once you have begun to talk about health behaviour with the patient it is important to assess how ready they are to change their health behaviour(s). Patients may feel willing but not actually have the confidence to change. Rollnick et al. (2007) propose adopting a curious approach to this rather than a question/answer manner.

> Nurse: 'OK John, because of what you initially said about nicotine gum, I'm unsure how you feel at the moment about stopping smoking and how important is it to you. Can we chat about this and then we can decide what to do next?'

From contemplation to preparation

> Patient: 'I am sick of being out of breath all the time and I know it's smoking that's causing it. Since you explained the different things that I could use to try to stop smoking, I may be able to give it another go. Especially if it will help me to lose weight as well. So, I have decided that I am definitely going to quit smoking after my holiday next month.'

> Nurse: 'That's great, and sometimes it's a good idea to have something to focus on. How about we set a date to follow this up when you get back from your holiday?'

It is important to remember that we can apply the model of behaviour change to any nursing setting and that patients may present to us at any stage in the cycle. For example, the patient and nurse scenario above could occur on a hospital ward, in an outpatient department or in a community setting. The key is that a follow-up opportunity has been discussed and arranged with all the necessary details communicated to those involved, so that when the patient returns both can continue to work through the process of moving the patient to the next stage. Once the patient has a real commitment to change then we need to discuss with them strategies for achieving goals and coping with relapses.

Jointly decide on goals and strategies to assist with relapse: set a SMART action plan

Action for change

Once the patient has a clearer view of the need for and benefits of behaviour change it is important to discuss how they are going to achieve their goal(s). One of the techniques used is motivational interviewing using SMART principles (Figure 15.4).

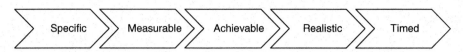

| Specific | Measurable | Achievable | Realistic | Timed |

Figure 15.4 SMART principles

In our case John has set a goal to quit smoking after his holiday and on returning has managed to cut down on the number of cigarettes he smokes per day. At present the prospect of a whole life without smoking may be overwhelming for John but a day without smoking may seem far more realistic. The key is to build up goals from the starting point.

Nurse: 'Hi, John, how was the holiday? Last time, you were considering stopping smoking when you got back. Shall we look at how we can help you with this?'

Patient: 'Well, I've managed to cut down but not given up completely. I think I need some help. What about nicotine patches. Will they help?'

Nurse: 'That's a good suggestion John. We need to enable you to reduce the number of cigarettes you smoke even further and it's a good idea to try patches. Let's set some small goals first so that it doesn't seem impossible. How about trying to cut down again by three cigarettes a day for the first week? Then, in 2 weeks' time, see how the patches help with a short-term goal of a whole day without smoking? Remember that as you reduce your smoking you will also see the benefits in your breathing, which will help you to get out and walk a bit more to increase your exercise'.

Notice the SMART principles in the example above. Decisions and goals agreed between the patient and the nurse are Specific, Measurable, Achievable, Realistic and Timed.

Maintenance

Devising coping strategies is important for success as many people have to cope with a number of difficulties until their new behaviour becomes the norm. Patients will adopt a variety of coping strategies and these should be explored with the patient as they may have very individual ideas and ways of doing this. Examples would include:

- changing routines
- finding substitutes.

Patient: 'I feel so much better. I haven't had a cigarette for 4 months now and that nicotine gum you suggested has really helped. Sometimes, though, I really crave one.'

Patient: 'I haven't smoked for over a year. It feels good when someone asks if I am a smoker and I say 'no'. I get tempted less and less and, if I do, I immediately get on with doing something to take my mind off it, like we discussed.'

Relapse

The experience patients undergo when changing health behaviour(s) can be life-changing for them. However, many do not exit the cycle the first time around and they relapse to their old unhealthy habits. Indeed, Prochaska and DiClemente found that, in the case of smokers, many had to take three journeys through the whole process before they were successful. It is important that we communicate to our patients their success and encouragement when things do not go to plan.

Patient: 'I was doing so well and then I got really stressed at work and a mate offered me a cigarette. Before I knew it, I'd smoked three and then bought a packet on the way home. I've failed again.'

Nurse: 'It's OK! It's inevitable that you'll slip back from time to time. We are all human! The important thing is to realise that you have been able to not smoke for such a long time, and you will be able to improve on this.'

The case scenario in this chapter has focused on working with an individual; however the same principles can be applied to working with groups or communities. Let's look at different settings and different skills we can apply.

Motivational interviewing

Motivational interviewing (MI) was developed by two psychologists, Miller and Rollnick, in the 1990s to tackle the motivation problems of people with alcohol dependency (Miller and Rollnick, 1995). There used to be an assumption among clinicians in this field that alcohol dependency treatment works for those who want to change, but if someone isn't motivated to stop drinking, no treatment in the world will work. Miller and Rollnick's interviewing technique for developing motivation was therefore quite a step forward. MI has been demonstrated to work in many trials now, including the Project MATCH study for alcohol dependency (Project MATCH Research Group, 1998), HIV and sexual health (Wolfers et al., 2009), increasing physical exercise (Frost et al., 2017) and improving mood of stroke survivors (Cheng et al., 2015). In general, it is often recommended for conditions that have poor treatment adherence such as addictions, bulimia, obesity and psychosis, but potentially it can be used for any situation where poor treatment adherence or engagement is an issue.

MI uses the principles of the Prochaska and DiClemente's Behaviour Change Model as illustrated above and fuses it with four principles taken from cognitive behavioural therapy (CBT) and Rogerian counselling. The nurse's intervention is pitched at the stage the patient is at in the model, and adopts two specific principles to target the motivation stage of the patient.

CBT: cognitive dissonance

Cognitive dissonance is a phenomenon identified in cognitive psychology whereby anyone feels psychologically uncomfortable when in a state of ambivalence; that is, when their behaviour and their values, attitudes or beliefs don't match. The principle of cognitive dissonance is that something has to change to relieve the person of that psychological discomfort; either they change their behaviour or they change their beliefs. For example, a woman who continues to drink excessively and discovers that her children are being harmed by her drinking behaviour will either have to stop drinking to stop feeling guilty or will develop beliefs and excuses for her behaviour, for example:

> 'It's an illness that I have no control over' or, 'my dad was a drinker and it didn't do me any harm when I was growing up'.

Using MI, the nurse targets the belief system to develop and enhance the discomfort, or 'dissonance'. This is called developing the **discrepancy** between behaviour and values.

Rogerian core principles of person-centred counselling

It sounds a bit cruel to just make someone feel uncomfortable about their behaviour but such therapeutic communication needs to be delivered in an ethical way; that is, person-centred. So, the relationship is based on Rogerian principles of expressing empathy and genuineness, working with the person to develop their self-efficacy and avoiding confrontation.

Boxes 15.2 and 15.3 outline the four principles of MI and specific techniques identified by Miller and Rollnick for practice application.

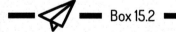 Box 15.2

Miller and Rollnick's four principles of MI in practice

1   Express empathy: use reflective listening skills to demonstrate understanding of the person's problems in a non-judgemental way.

(Continued)

2   Develop discrepancy: between the person's deeply held values and their current behaviour.
3   Roll with the resistance that inevitably occurs: don't be confrontational or get into an argument.
4   Support and promote self-efficacy: help the person to believe they can effect change for themselves.

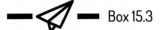 **Box 15.3**

Specific techniques in MI

- Strive to understand the person's point of view and experiences, and make it clear to them that you accept their unique condition.
- Focus on statements that encourage change and don't focus on negative or 'stuck' statements such as 'I can't change – there's no point trying'.
- Ask questions that elicit self-statements of problem recognition and desire to change, such as 'if you stopped drinking now, what would your life be like in 5 years' time?'
- Match your questions to the person's stage of change – don't jump ahead of the patient.
- Constantly refer back to the patient's ability to choose their own path.

Knowledge link Chapter 7 gives a fuller description of Rogerian principles and CBT, and Chapter 12 outlines MI in chronic illness.

Anyone in healthcare can use MI skills when faced with patients with poor compliance and poor prognosis. Often, such patients are seen as 'heart-sink' patients, because nurses become frustrated trying to persuade them to change their behaviour. Such patients may be good candidates for MI.

Let's look at some of the new skills mentioned above. There are examples of others in Chapter 7. The techniques must of course be based on an empathetic and co-operative style of relationship-building.

How to develop discrepancy

A person with a serious health problem due to their behaviour or lifestyle is often in denial about the reality of their situation. They have already closed their minds to the facts and developed defences such as a set of beliefs that protect them from feeling uncomfortable. Just telling someone won't get very far as they have been told enough times before. It is up to the interviewer to highlight the reality of their situation. We can refer to some of the negative points whenever the opportunity presents, and create those opportunities by getting the person to state them for themselves. This is called eliciting a **self-statement**. See the example in Box 15.4.

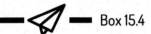 Box 15.4

A sexual health nurse is interviewing a sex industry worker

Patient: 'I would like to know whether I'm HIV-positive or not.'

Nurse: 'What's stopping you?'

Patient: 'Well, because they might say I am HIV positive!'

Nurse: 'And what would be bad about that?'

Patient:
(laughs) 'Well, it would mean I'm going to die wouldn't it?'

Notice the nurse gets the patient to make the statement about this fear herself, even though the answer is easy to anticipate. That way, the person is 'owning' her own values rather than having them thrust upon her in a confronting way. This style of questioning is called Socratic questioning, where the nurse persists in asking even obvious questions in order to get the person to make the obvious statements of fact or belief themselves.

Knowledge link Chapter 4 also addresses Socratic questioning.

Roll with resistance and avoid argumentation

Direct advice and confrontation with someone who is ambivalent about change will simply create resistance and defensiveness. See Box 15.5.

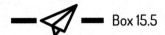 Box 15.5

Creating resistance

Nurse: 'Have you thought about cutting down on your smoking? It will help reduce your blood pressure.'

Patient: 'Yes, I've tried but frankly, I enjoy smoking. It helps me relax and that probably reduces my blood pressure too.'

Nurse: 'But you could relax in other ways. In the long term your blood pressure will be reduced if you stop smoking.'

Patient: 'Yes, but ... '

This interviewer has got into an argumentative dialogue with this patient and the patient is now resisting with the 'yes, but ... ' position.

Look at the next example (Box 15.6).

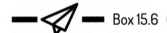 Box 15.6

Rolling with resistance

Nurse: 'I guess you've tried cutting down your smoking?'

Patient: 'Oh yes, but as soon as I feel stressed or go out socially, I want a cigarette.'

Nurse: 'What do you think makes you smoke in those situations?' (avoiding a confrontational question)

Patient: 'Just habit, I suppose, but when I'm stressed, I don't care about my health.'

Nurse: (in response to the negative stance by the patient) 'I can see on those occasions it is hard. Let's look at when you find it easier.'

Notice how the nurse has spotted that they are about to fall into an oppositional relationship, so the nurse agrees with the patient about it being hard (because it is!) and moves towards talking about success instead of failure. This will also highlight the patient's sense of self-efficacy – what they *can* do.

So, the relationship is about 'being on the same side' as the patient in making changes rather than being in a professional–patient relationship and resorting to advice and persuasion. It has been established for a while that treatment dropout is higher when the professional adopts a dictatorial style (Stott and Pill, 1990).

Resistance in the patient can be spotted by the development of:

- arguing
- interrupting
- denying
- ignoring.

The key to dealing with resistance is to recognise it and move away from the topic or shift the focus, ensuring that the patient knows it is about their own choice. We can then go back to the topic once we feel that the time is right and the patient is much more open to discussion. Rollnick et al. (2007) offer a useful checklist that we can adapt for nursing to check that we are getting it right:

- The nurse is speaking slowly.
- The patient is doing much of the talking – about behaviour change.
- The nurse is listening carefully, only directing the interview at appropriate stages.
- The patient is 'working hard' and asking the nurse for advice and information.
- It is as if the nurse and the patient are putting the pieces of a jigsaw together to reveal the full picture.

Support self-efficacy

The main aim of MI is to promote the patient's perception of their own abilities to make changes. A good strategy to adopt when meeting any resistance is to acknowledge and empathise with the patient's view and focus on the achievement the patient has made, even if it seems small. A resistant patient turning up for a clinic appointment is often a positive sign of motivation and hope, and can be explored. See Box 15.7.

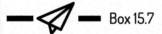 Box 15.7

Encouraging self-efficacy

Patient: 'I can't alter the way I am. I'm just fat and that's that.'

Interviewer: 'You sound really fed up about it, but I think you are already making changes by coming here. You've made a very positive start.'

Notice the nurse emphasises that the patient has done something positive, implying that the patient is already making choices about change. The nurse might have emphasised how much attending clinic will help the patient – but that takes the power to change away from the patient, suggesting that it is the *clinic* that will make the difference. Instead, the nurse gives the message that the patient will make the difference by choosing to attend the clinic and use the help on offer.

Brief intervention

With pre-contemplative patients, it is hard to get as far as even discussing the problem without meeting instant resistance and disinterest. However, there is another evidence-based technique we can employ which aims to move someone towards contemplation of change. This is called brief intervention therapy (BIT).

Brief intervention aims to raise the patient's awareness of the problem and reduce any misconceptions. It adopts a similar strategy to MI by avoiding confrontation and helping the patient 'own' their beliefs by eliciting self-statements. Look at the example in Box 15.8.

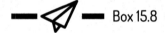 Box 15.8

Brief intervention

An underage teenage girl presents at the emergency department with alcohol poisoning. She indulges in heavy binge-drinking most weekends. Her understanding of her risk is epitomised by her statements: 'Everyone I know drinks like I do, there's nothing wrong with them. I'm young and fit, my body can cope.'

Nurse: 'I see you are due for a liver scan in a bit. Do you know what that's for?'

Patient: 'Just to check that my liver's OK I guess.'

Nurse: (looking serious) 'Well, it's a bit more than that really. There may be liver damage, judging by your level of alcohol intake. A female of your age is particularly vulnerable to liver damage.'

The nurse is being quite dramatic but not unrealistically so and is not 'preaching'. The message being given is that this person in particular is at specific risk of liver damage. This indirectly challenges the patient's existing beliefs of being invulnerable at her age.

Brief intervention is about sowing seeds of doubt or hope, giving people 'food for thought' and making even a small change to how the person views their situation and behaviour. When someone presents with an acute problem, it is very often a good opportunity to highlight the reality of their behaviour. However, it is more effective if it is personalised – the message is: it is *you* who are in hospital/clinic, *you* who are having immediate treatment and *you* who has chosen this course of action.

Another strategy in BIT is to elicit a statement about what the person would like to change if they could. A person who believes they are predestined to fail can still have dreams or have a wish list. See Box 15.9 for a real example of BIT with a female heroin user, instilling hope rather than hopelessness.

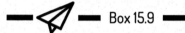 Box 15.9

Working with a drug-using sex worker

Nurse: 'If you had a magic wand, what would you change?'

Patient: 'Oh, I'd go back in time and not start taking heroin.'

Nurse: 'If you could do that, what would you have done instead?'

Patient: 'I'd have gone to college and perhaps been a nurse or something, instead of prostitution.'

Nurse: 'Going to college sounds like something you could do in the future.'

Patient: 'But I've ruined my life already.'

Nurse: 'Not yet. You're still alive. Some of your friends aren't. They have ruined their lives. You haven't.'

With BIT, the seeds sown often need to be left to take effect. The health professional has no control over what people do with the intervention given during the short opportunity that presents. Evidence of effectiveness of BIT (O'Donnell et al., 2014) indicates that it may be the first prompt that gets someone to think about things, seek more information and perhaps approach health services for support.

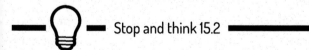 Stop and think 15.2

Test yourself on what you have learned about MI and BIT by trying this multiple choice questionnaire.

(Continued)

1   MI:
    a   Is about confronting the person about their health risk behaviour
    b   Is only relevant for drug and alcohol problems
    c   Requires the health professional to be specially trained
    d   Should be delivered with a person-centred approach
    e   Was found to be less effective than ordinary CBT by the Project MATCH study.

2   Strategies in MI include:
    a   Directly challenging the patient's beliefs
    b   Agreeing with the patient at all times
    c   Looking for arguments
    d   Taking on the role of the expert professional
    e   Looking out for resistance.

3   BIT:
    a   Is a form of psychotherapy
    b   Is complicated to deliver
    c   Aims to elicit negative statements from the patient
    d   Aims to elicit hopeful statements from the patient
    e   Aims to tell the patient their beliefs are wrong.

4   In practising MI or BIT, the practitioner needs to:
    a   Encourage the patient to make choices
    b   Challenge the patient's defences
    c   Tell the patient when they are wrong
    d   Advise the patient how to behave more healthily
    e   Teach the patient how to change.

Answers: 1 (d); 2 (e); 3 (d); 4 (a).

Conclusion

Modern nursing is not just about caring for the sick patient. Nurses are now health promoters and should help patients adopt healthier lifestyles. To do this, we need the communication skills that encourage people to engage in healthier behaviour. Using theory to guide our communication enables us to work with patients in a logical way and to plan interventions with them that target their individual needs. As nurses, we need to be aware of the impact that our position can have on our patient's ability to consider healthy behaviours and use this in a way that facilitates and encourages behaviour change. This process requires effective communication skills if we want to achieve positive outcomes for our patients.

....**RECOMMENDED READING**

Miller, W.R. and Rollnick, S. (2012) *Motivational Interviewing: Helping People Change (Applications of Motivational Interviewing)* (3rd edn). New York, Guilford Press.
Scriven, A. (2017) *Ewles & Simnett's Promoting Health: A Practical Guide* (7th edn). London, Elsevier.

....**REFERENCES**

Armstrong, S., Anderson, M., Le, E. and Nguyen, L. (2009) Application of the Health Belief Model to bariatric surgery. *Gastroenterology Nursing*, 32(3), 171–178.
Browes, S. (2006) Health psychology and sexual health assessment. *Nursing Standard*, 21(5), 35–39.
Cheng, D., Qu, Z., Huang, J., Xiao, Y., Luo, H. and Wang, J. (2015) Motivational interviewing for improving recovery after stroke. *Cochrane Database of Systematic Reviews*, 6, CD011398.
Coulson, N.S., Ferguson, M.A., Henshaw. H. and Heffernan, E. (2016) Applying theories of health behaviour and change to hearing health research: time for a new approach. *International Journal of Audiology*, 55, S99–S104.
Frost, H., Campbell, P., Maxwell, M., O'Carroll, R.E., Dombrowski, S.U., Williams, B., Cheyne, H., Coles, E. and Pollock, A. (2017) Effectiveness of Motivational Interviewing on adult behaviour change in health and social care settings: a systematic review of reviews. *PLoS ONE*, 13(10), e0204890.
Gilliver, M., Beach, E.F. and Williams, W. (2015) Changing beliefs about leisure noise: using health promotion models to investigate young people's engagement with, and attitudes towards, hearing health. *International Journal of Audiology*, 54(4), 211–219.
Langley, E.L., Wootton, B.M. and Grieve, R. (2018) The utility of the health belief model variables in predicting help-seeking intention for anxiety disorders. *Australian Psychologist*, 53(4), 291–301.
Luquis, R. and Kensinger, W. (2019) Applying the Health Belief Model to assess prevention services among young adults. *International Journal of Health Promotion and Education*, 57(1), 37–47.
Medina-Shepherd, R. and Kleier, J. (2010) Spanish translation and adaptation of Victoria Champion's Health Belief Model Scales for breast cancer screening – mammography. *Cancer Nursing*, 33(2), 93–101.
Miller, W.R. and Rollnick, S. (1995) *Motivational Interviewing: Preparing People to Change*. New York, Guilford Press.
Noushirvani, S. and Mansouri, A. (2018) Comparison of the effect of two educational interventions based on Pender's Health Promotion Model and Health Belief Model on the quality of life in Type 2 diabetic patients. *Journal of Diabetic Nursing*, 6(1), 398–407.
O'Donnell, A., Wallace, P. and Kaner, E. (2014) From efficacy to effectiveness and beyond: what next for brief interventions in primary care? *Frontiers in Psychiatry*, 5(113), 1–8.
Prochaska, J.O. and DiClemente, C.C. (1986) Toward a comprehensive model of change. In W. Miller and N. Heather (eds), *Addictive Behaviors: Processes of Change* (pp. 3–27). New York, Plenum Press.
Prochaska, J.O., Norcross, J.C. and DiClemente, C.C. (1994) *Changing for Good*. New York, Willam Marrow and Company.

Project MATCH Research Group (1998) Matching alcoholism treatments to patient heterogeneity: Project MATCH three-year drinking outcomes. *Alcohol Clinical Experimental Research*, 22, 1300–1311.

Rollnick, S., Mason, P. and Butler, C. (2007) *Health Behaviour Change. A Guide for Practitioners*. Edinburgh, Churchill Livingstone.

Rosenstock, I. (1974) The HBM and preventative health behaviour. *Health Education Monographs*, 2, 354–368.

Schofield, I., Kerr, S. and Tolson, D. (2007) An exploration of the smoking-related health beliefs of older people with chronic obstructive pulmonary disease. *Journal of Clinical Nursing*, 16(9), 1726–1735.

Scriven, A. (2017) *Ewles & Simnett's Promoting Health: A Practical Guide* (7th edn). London, Elsevier.

Stott, N. and Pill, R. (1990) 'Advise yes, dictate no'. Patients' views on health promotion in the consultation. *Family Practice*, 7(2), 125–131.

Wolfers, M., de Wit, J., Hospers, H., Richardus, J. and de Zwart, O. (2009) Effects of a short individually tailored counselling session for HIV prevention in gay and bisexual men receiving hepatitis B vaccination. *BMC Public Health*, 9, 255.

SIXTEEN
COMMUNICATION FOR PERSONAL AND PROFESSIONAL DEVELOPMENT: PRE-REGISTRATION AND POST-REGISTRATION

LUCY WEBB

.... THIS CHAPTER WILL HELP YOU TO:

- Maintain your portfolio for personal and professional development
- Use professional support structures to learn from experience in practice
- Use professional support structures to develop self–awareness

Introduction

Right from the beginning of Chapter 1, we emphasised that communication is a key practice area in the NMC's standards of proficiency for professional nurses (NMC, 2018a). During a pre-registration or nursing associate course, students are exposed to increasingly complex practice challenges that help develop levels of competency. With each term and year, you will be building on existing knowledge towards the competency required of a nurse on the NMC register. However, development does not stop there! The NMC *Code*

(NMC, 2018b) requires all registered nurses to continue to develop and update skills and knowledge, and be able to demonstrate engagement with continued learning to revalidate their registration.

This chapter aims to give you a brief introduction to some of the ways in which you can engage with this process as a student, and to continue to develop your communication skills when qualified.

Rationale for continuing personal and professional development

Healthcare professionals working in the UK, especially in the NHS, need to comply with the clinical governance for health service delivery. This is a system of standards which providers of healthcare must adhere to in order to ensure high-quality and safe care (RCN, 2018a). This applies to service providers (such as hospital managers) and all clinical staff members, and is focused on five key themes (see Box 16.1).

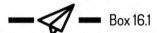 Box 16.1

The five key themes of clinical governance

1   Patient focus: how services are based on patient needs
2   Information focus: how information is used
3   Quality improvement: how standards are reviewed and attained
4   Staff focus: how staff are developed
5   Leadership: how improvement efforts are planned.

(RCN, 2018b)

We can list some examples of good communication skills under each theme (see Box 16.2).

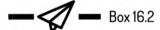 Box 16.2

Clinical governance themes with examples

1   Patient focus: listening skills, emotional intelligence, empathy, developing a trusting relationship, liaising with informal carers, advocating for patients to colleagues
2   Information focus: informing colleagues, keeping up-to-date and accurate records
3   Quality improvement: reporting and escalating concerns, leadership and teamwork

4   Staff focus: continued professional development, mentoring and supervising junior staff and students

5   Leadership: role-modelling, supervision, team management, emotional intelligence applied to staff members.

As a student entering the nursing profession, the emphasis on autonomous practice, accountability, lifelong learning and professional development may seem at times at odds with your experience of the culture in practice. Mackintosh (2006) found that some students became disillusioned when encountering nurses in practice who were uncaring or unprofessional. These students found that some nurses had lost their commitment to nursing and it had become just a routine job. Clinical governance and the focus on personal and professional development aims to overcome the problems of this depreciation of skills and attitudes among trained professionals who can become unmotivated and outdated in their practice and, consequently, deliver a poor standard of care. Following the inquiry into governance failings of Mid Staffordshire NHS Foundation Trust, the Francis Report (Francis, 2013) identified many key issues that related to poor communication:

a   no systems in place for clinical quality or staff monitoring
b   information gathering was 'inept' and coding 'dreadful'
c   failure of information-sharing between agencies
d   failure to build a positive culture, in nursing in particular
e   staff not embracing the importance of clinical governance
f   no culture of self-analysis
g   little analysis of complaints or incidents
h   out-of-date risk register.

While these are organisational issues, you can see how individual practitioners at this hospital were failing to deliver the principles of communication skills on an individual level – leadership, record-keeping, information-sharing, self-development and awareness – thus escalating concerns.

As nurses need to become more autonomous professionals, modern nurse training aims to ensure we can maintain good quality professional standards throughout our careers. We also need to demonstrate we have done this through continuing professional development (CPD). As a student, you may be maintaining a learning portfolio to record and monitor your progress. When you are qualified, you will need to continue this practice to collect evidence of your CPD for revalidation. We will look at portfolios and revalidation later.

Firstly, let's look at the two key mechanisms that help students to engage in both professional and personal development: the relationship between the student and practice facilitator and the use and practice of reflection.

The student–practice supervisor relationship

A practice supervisor (sometimes still referred to as a mentor) will be a registered health professional allocated to students in the practice setting. They will provide learning experiences that enable the student to meet their learning outcomes in practice. The supervisor does not necessarily do the 'teaching' in practice but will facilitate learning opportunities, ensure the student practises safely and give feedback and encouragement for the student to learn and develop skills (NMC, 2018c). The effectiveness of this role relies on a positive working relationship between the student and the supervisor (Houghton, 2016). Hence, a supervisor has to be a student's support and make judgements about the student's progress and learning needs, as well as being a practising nurse.

Students have described a good supervisor as friendly, patient, accessible and, in particular, nurturing (Wilkes, 2006). Houghton (2016) suggests that an effective supervisor is, among many things, enthusiastic, approachable, organised and a good communicator. Supervisors are expected to understand the student's experience but, equally, if the student can understand the supervisor's experience, a relationship of partnership and mutual respect is more likely to develop.

Hart (2010) suggests that students have a wealth of learning opportunities on every placement but need to engage with the staff available to get the most out of these situations. She advises that you take every opportunity you can to learn while in practice. Show enthusiasm to learn and push yourself forward. It is easy for busy supervisors to forget you are there and that you need to see what they are doing. You may need to be diplomatic rather than be a pest, but you will experience so much more by being proactive!

We can see that a good student–supervisor relationship requires competent communication skills on both sides. As a student, you have a responsibility to seek learning opportunities. To take full advantage of them, a trusting and mutually respectful relationship will help facilitate your learning and overall experience in practice. You should deploy professional relating and communication skills from the outset of your training.

Reflective practice

This brings us on to reflective practice, which is a vital component of personal and professional development for the student and the qualified nurse. Reflection relies on good communication skills and aids development of the underpinning skills of self-awareness, assertiveness, confidence and personal development. Reflection is acknowledged as a key component in helping the practitioner to change perspective and develop new insights. Reflection on practice leads to action and change (Johns, 1995), but it is also a skill in itself that needs development and leads to 'reflection as a way of being' (Johns, 2005:6). See Box 16.3 for an example of Johns' model of reflection and the five cue questions that aid your reflection on an episode.

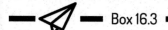 Box 16.3

Johns' model of reflection: five cue questions

Reflection

1   What was I trying to achieve and what are the consequences?

Influencing factors

2   What things, like internal/external/knowledge, affected my decision-making?
3   Could I have dealt with it better?
4   What other choices did I have and what were the consequences?

Learning

5   What will change because of this experience, how did I feel about the experience and how has this experience changed my ways of knowing?

We can distinguish between reflection as a tool and as a skill by considering:

*   reflection on practice: learning from practice experiences (reflection on action)
*   reflection in practice: applying reflective skills during practice (reflection in action).

Reflection on practice (reflection on action)

Reflection *on* practice is reflection following a nursing event and aids the nurse to consider actions, decisions and dilemmas arising from practice experience, and to consider them through analysis and evaluation. There are a host of reflective practice tools and methods that can be used for this purpose which extend from directive guidance for the novice reflector to internalisation and insight and self-directed reflection for the expert reflector (Morgan and Johns, 2005). You may be familiar with some of the more directive methods in the list below:

a   Reflective diary: facilitates later reflection on thoughts, feelings and acts written in the context of practice. It communicates the nurse's ability to consider one's practice and seek to improve it.

b   Significant event record: an account of a specific event reviewed historically for insights from the event.

c   Supervision: guided refection in dialogue, often using Socratic dialogue from the supervisor to explore meaning of experiences and modify the reflector's thinking and knowledge.

d   Structured reflective models: for example, Gibbs' reflective cycle, Johns' model of reflection; two common reflective models that take the reflector through a series of questions to discover new insights on events.

e   Intuitive reflection: on-the-spot or later critical thinking without specific tools, sleeping on problems, brainstorming and mind-mapping.

The key aspect of reflection on practice is opening up a personal dialogue with yourself regarding a particular incident, event or situation that has occurred. This is a form of communication with yourself, using tools or mechanisms to engage in thinking. Hamilton and Martin (2007) suggested a framework to improve nurses' communications with patients (see Box 16.4).

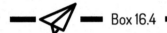 Box 16.4

Hamilton and Martin's framework: reflection on practice questions

*   What interventions or skills did I use?
*   What was the purpose of using these skills?
*   What was my goal?
*   Did I achieve what I set out to achieve?
*   What would I do differently?

(Hamilton and Martin, 2007)

Hamilton and Martin suggest that this reflection should focus on the effects of your communication skills during the interaction. For example, you may want to examine your ability to empathise, to convey health promotion information or to reassure a patient. This way, you can specify the skill you want to develop.

Reflection in practice (reflection in action)

Reflection *in* practice can be described as the skill of reflection applied in practice – at the time of practice (Johns, 1995; Todd, 2005). The practice of reflection *on* practice develops the nurse's ability to think objectively and form a different perspective about practice and professional development issues. Reflection *in* practice is putting those reflection skills to use when in a practice situation. In considering communication skills, you may have become aware that, for example, in a multi-disciplinary team meeting you tend to lack assertiveness and need to take opportunities to put your views across. In your next multi-disciplinary team meeting, you could assess the situation objectively, perhaps finding you have not stated your case well, have used passive speech (as in 'I think it might be a good idea to ... ') rather than active speech (as in 'It is a good idea to ... ') and need to act assertively to better present your view to your colleagues.

Reflection is an important aspect of personal and professional development for healthcare professionals and has long been seen as an effective way to develop skills in practice (Schon, 1983; Casement, 1985). It is included in this book from the perspective of communication because, without good communication skills, we could not engage in reflection through writing or dialogue.

Professional skills development: 'on-the-job' CPD

Clinical supervision

Clinical supervision is traditionally practised more in some fields of nursing and midwifery than others. It is commonly found in mental health nursing, and has even been a statutory requirement in midwifery until recently, but appears rarely practised in generic adult nursing. The NMC no longer gives advice on clinical supervision as it is commonly agreed that it should be part of localised processes of training rather than incorporated into formal clinical governance. That said, nurses and midwives in certain fields of care may encounter forms of clinical supervision in their practice.

Evidence for effectiveness for clinical supervision is quite weak, although this may be because of a lack of good-quality research more than there being evidence against clinical supervision (Pollock et al., 2017). One clear factor from the evidence, however, is how *effective* clinical supervision is depends on how it is carried out (White and Winstanley, 2010).

Good clinical supervision requires good skills of communication by supervisor and supervisee. Effective supervision needs the supervisor and supervisee to develop a working relationship that encourages discussion. Butterworth et al. (2008) suggest that clinical supervision has many benefits but also some failings. As a CPD tool, it can increase the supervisee's confidence and self-awareness, reduce their sense of isolation, improve their work–life balance and increase personal growth and coping. It also facilitates knowledge transfer to less experienced practitioners and helps bridge the theory–practice gap.

Butterworth et al. (2008) also point out that effective clinical supervision demands organisational support to overcome problems of tokenism or lack of staff engagement. Poorly practised supervision can create resistance among staff, leading to suspicion, lack of disclosure and a feeling that it is just a management tool. It could also be destructive by becoming a means with which to air grievances, and creating an 'us-and-them' division between management and staff.

Proctor's model of clinical supervision

A key contributor to the development of clinical supervision in nursing, Brigid Proctor (1986), suggested three functional components to clinical supervision:

1   Normative: providing a structure to practice supervision, meeting and addressing professional ethics requirements and ensuring professional responsibility.
2   Restorative: providing support to staff, enabling personal growth, professionalism, confidence and problem-solving skills, and producing higher staff morale.
3   Formative: providing educative and skills development among staff, sharing of knowledge and experience and contributing to the incorporation of theory and practice.

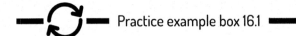 Practice example box 16.1

Clinical supervision

A nurse brought a concern to her supervisor regarding a patient in palliative care with severe dementia. The patient's relatives wanted him to receive communion from the hospital priest. The patient's history suggested he had lost interest in practising his religion, although the family were practising Catholics. The nurse was unsure who she should be an advocate for: the relatives or the patient. In discussing this case, the supervisor and supervisee explored the issues of consent and advocacy and decided that the patient would consent if able as the relatives would be comforted. Additionally, there was no evidence to suggest that he would object, while he may even feel comforted at this stage in his life. The nurse felt confident about deciding to facilitate the communion and understood more clearly the role of advocate and issues of consent and mental capacity.

Practice example box 16.1 provides a real-life example of a supervision scenario. Firstly, this formalised supervision provision complies with Proctor's normative component in that supervision was organised and available to the nurse, providing a vehicle for addressing professional ethics and the nurse's accountability. Secondly, it illustrates Proctor's restorative function of supervision whereby the nurse had moved from having doubts about her practice to feeling confident with her own accountability for the decision made; the nurse had been provided with knowledgeable support and guidance. Thirdly, we can see Proctor's formative component in this example whereby the nurse has developed professionally by extending her knowledge and experience.

Proctor's model provides clarity and boundaries to the relationship of supervisor–supervisee in that it defines the aims of clinical supervision. As outlined earlier, poorly delivered supervision detracts from these functions.

One problem identified by Cutliffe and Proctor (1998) is that supervision relies both on a skilled supervisor and also a supervisee who knows how to use the supervision offered. Lack of understanding of clinical supervision can lead to mistrust and resistance; hence Cutliffe and Proctor (1998) suggest that nurses need to be socialised into receiving and using supervision even during training. Bond and Holland (1998) suggest that the supervisee should understand the supervisee role and should be fully engaged and committed to supervision. Supervision cannot meet Proctor's aims, arguably, when the supervision is imposed by management on an unwilling workforce.

Bond and Holland (1998) suggest that the supervisee should:

a   have an active part in selecting the supervisor
b   have adequate preparation for the session
c   develop skills in reflective practice
d   identify topics for discussion
e   help set ground rules.

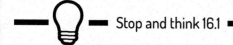 Stop and think 16.1

Next time you are in a practice placement, find out what clinical supervision processes are in place. There may not be an identified or formal system for clinical supervision, but find out how nurses engage in reflection and learning from practice episodes. Do you think these methods meet the requirements of personal and professional development as outlined in the evidence for good practice here? What would improve the engagement in personal and professional development?

Reflection point 16.1 answer: you might have considered whether nurses are engaging in guided reflection or rely on informal self-directed and insightful reflection. Also, are there any clinical supervision structures in place? If not, how do nurses consider clinical issues from their practice, and are these methods adequate?

Self-directed skills development

While you may have learning resources available in practice provided by your employer, there is still a need for nurses to initiate their own professional development and there's no reason why you shouldn't find your own ways to learn. McCluskey et al. (2011) found from a scoping study among Scottish healthcare practitioners that they mostly preferred to develop communication skills in the practice setting rather than a classroom. Approaches such as reflection and clinical supervision are helpful but the practitioners in McCluskey et al.'s study preferred approaches such as:

a   self-review and reflection tools in a checklist format
b   facilitated scenario work and role play
c   feedback from patients
d   peer observation of practice
e   training that is focused on general skills rather than specialist skills
f   use of technology for self-directed learning (DVDs, e-learning, video) feedback training.

However, as suggested by Hamilton and Martin (2007), communication skills development in the practice setting also requires commitment and willingness among teams and management. Therefore, it is likely that approaches which include whole-team inclusion will also support individual practitioners to develop their skills.

Continuing professional development and communication skills

Revalidation

The NMC requires all registered nurses and midwives to revalidate their registration every 3 years (NMC, 2017). The revalidation process is a way of ensuring that practitioners are keeping up to date with evidence-based practice, and, particularly, are continuing to engage with the NMC *Code* and are continuing to practise safely and effectively.

As part of **revalidation**, you will need to keep a record to demonstrate that you have completed a minimum of 450 hours of practice and 35 hours of CPD. Twenty of those CPD hours must be participatory; that is, training in which you have personally interacted with other professionals, such as in a group learning situation. Your communication skills development can count as CPD. In the next section, we will suggest ways you can collect and archive your learning.

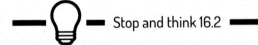 Stop and think 16.2

Visit www.youtube.com/watch?v=mcAn6MrSBDk&feature=youtu.be to see the NMC's own video on revalidation for further information on this process. You can also go to the NMC's website to access their information guides and booklets (see also the Further reading list).

Portfolios

As a student nurse, you will hopefully have become familiar with keeping a learning portfolio that is a record of your progress through your training. Before you file it away when you qualify and think you need never see it again, bear in mind you will need to continue to keep a record of your CPD to revalidate your registration with the NMC. As described above, you will need to keep evidence of your CPD and a portfolio is an ideal way to do this.

A portfolio is recommended by the NMC to record evidence that you have met the requirements for revalidation of your registration. Your portfolio can take whatever format that suits you – either a paper version or e-portfolio – but you will of course need to adhere to the NMC *Code* regarding confidentiality and store only anonymised data in the portfolio. You will not need to share it with the NMC, either: you only need to discuss the evidence with someone who will act as the confirmer of your revalidation evidence. This will be a registered professional, perhaps someone at work, a supervisor, colleague or independent assessor.

Your portfolio and communication skills development

The evidence of communication skills development in your portfolio could include certificates of any relevant training or course/conference attendance, reflective accounts from practice or clinical supervision and records of experiences you may have had as part of your work or outside of work that contributed to your skills development. For instance, a volunteering role that tested your public speaking or teaching abilities would count as a learning experience that developed your professional skills. The key information you need to collect is listed by the NMC guide to revalidation (see Further reading list):

a the CPD method used (such as self-learning, online learning or training course)
b a brief description of the topic and how it relates to your practice
c the dates the CPD activity was undertaken
d the number of hours and participatory hours
e identification of the part of the *Code* most relevant to the CPD
f evidence of the CPD activity (e.g. record of attendance, signed affirmation from a supervisor or trainer, or written reflection).

Fortunately, the NMC has made this revalidation evidence collection and recording easy by providing templates for the different elements of the process. You will find these templates or links to them in the NMC guide to revalidation in the Further reading list.

The Further reading list in this chapter gives a link to the NMC's guide to revalidation (NMC, 2019). Alternatively, search NMC revalidation for links to their information.

Conclusion

This chapter has illustrated a very important element of nursing that is dependent on communication skills: CPD. We have outlined just two of the many ways that you can engage in and demonstrate your skills development. You will already have experienced reflective practice as a student nurse and may also have been exposed to clinical supervision in practice – at least observing its function among nursing teams. Reflective practices are described as essential tools to support personal and professional development. They aid the nurse to learn from practice (reflection on practice) and apply reflective skills in practice (reflection in practice). So, like communication skills, reflection is a skill to be developed and understood and a tool for developing the skills of objectivity and application of learning in practice.

Clinical supervision, on the other hand, is a tool we can use to *facilitate* personal and professional development. It is a method for developing the underpinning communication skills of self-awareness, assertiveness, confidence and even self-esteem as part of our professional identity. However, both reflection and supervision can be enacted either through tokenism – going through the motions – or by quality engagement with CPD. It is the professional nurse's responsibility not only to demonstrate CPD but also to engage meaningfully with the processes of CPD to enhance practice. Once you have qualified, you will be expected to seek out opportunities to engage in CPD and demonstrate your development through revalidation. Learning doesn't stop when you qualify. It could be said that it has only just started!

FURTHER READING

Johns, C. and Freshwater, D. (eds) (2005) *Transforming Nursing Through Reflective Practice* (2nd edn). Oxford, Blackwell Publishing.

Lidster, J. and Wakefield, S (2018) *Student Practice Supervision and Assessment: A Guide for NMC Nurses and Midwives.* London, SAGE Publications.

NMC (2018) *Revalidation: Your Step-by-Step Guide Through the Process.* http://revalidation. nmc.org.uk/download-resources/guidance-and-information.html.

NMC (2019) *Welcome to Revalidation.* http://revalidation.nmc.org.uk/welcome-to-revalidation/.

REFERENCES

Bond, M. and Holland, S. (1998) *Skills of Clinical Supervision for Nurses: A Practical Guide for Supervisees, Clinical Supervisors and Managers.* Buckingham, Open University Press.

Butterworth, T., Bell, L., Jackson, C. and Pajnkihar, M. (2008) Wicked spell or magic bullet? A review of the clinical supervision literature 2001–2007. *Nurse Education Today,* 28, 264–272.

Casement, P. (1985) *On Learning from the Patient.* New York, Guildford Press.

Cutliffe, J. and Proctor, B. (1998) An alternative training approach to clinical supervision: 1. *British Journal of Nursing*, 7(5), 280–285.

Francis, R. (2013) *Mid Staffordshire NHS Trust Public Inquiry*. https://webarchive. nationalarchives.gov.uk/20150407084231/http://www.midstaffspublicinquiry.com/report.

Hamilton, L. and Martin, D. (2007) Clinical development: a framework for effective communication skills. *Nursing Times*. www.nursingtimes.net/clinical-archive/leadership/ clinical-development-a-framework-for-effective-communication-skills/296359.article.

Hart, S. (2010) *Nursing: Study and Placement Learning Skills*. Oxford, Oxford University Press.

Houghton, T. (2016) Establishing effective working relationships. *Nursing Standard*, 30(26), 41–48.

Johns, C. (1995) Framing learning through reflection within Carper's ways of knowing in nursing. *Journal of Advanced Nursing*, 22, 226–234.

Johns, C. (2005) Expanding the gates of perception. In C. Johns and D. Freshwater (eds), *Transforming Nursing Through Reflective Practice* (2nd edn; pp. 1–12). Oxford, Blackwell Publishing.

Mackintosh, C. (2006) Caring: the socialisation of pre-registration student nurses. A longitudinal qualitative descriptive study. *International Journal of Nursing Studies*, 43, 953–962.

McCluskey, S., Heywood, S. and Fitzgerald, N. (2011) *How Healthcare Professionals in Scotland Develop their Communication Skills, Attitudes and Behaviours. An Independent Report for NHS Education Scotland*. www.new.scot.nhs.uk/media/547484/long-term_conditions- communication-and-human-relationships/pdf.

Morgan, R. and Johns, C. (2005) The beast and the star: resolving contradictions within everyday practice. In C. Johns and D. Freshwater (eds), *Transforming Nursing Through Reflective Practice* (2nd edn; pp. 114–128). Oxford, Blackwell Publishing.

NMC (2017) *How to Revalidate with the NMC: Requirements for Renewing your Registration*. London, Nursing and Midwifery Council.

NMC (2018a) *Future Nurse: Standards of Proficiency for Registered Nurses*. www.nmc.org.uk/ globalassets/sitedocuments/education-standards/future-nurse-proficiencies.pdf.

NMC (2018b) *The Code: Professional Standards of Practice and Behaviour for Nurses, Midwives and Nursing Associates*. www.nmc.org.uk/standards/code/.

NMC (2018c) *Practice Supervision: Guides*. London, Nursing and Midwifery Council.

Pollock, A., Campbell, P., Deery, R., Fleming, M., Rankin, J., Sloan, G. and Cheyne, H. (2017) A systematic review of evidence relating to clinical supervision for nurses, midwives and allied health professionals. *Journal of Advanced Nursing*, 73(8), 1825–1837.

Proctor, B. (1986) Supervision: a co-operative exercise in accountability. In M. Marken and M. Payn (eds), *Enabling and Ensuring* (pp. 21–23). Leicester, Leicester National Youth Bureau and Council for Education and Training in Youth & Community Work.

RCN (2018a) *Clinical Governance*. www.rcn.org.uk/clinical-topics/clinical-governance.

RCN (2018b) *Clinical Governance: Five Key Themes*. www.rcn.org.uk/clinical-topics/clinical- governance/five-key-themes.

Schon, D. (1983) *Educating the Reflective Practitioner*. London, Jossey Bass.

Todd, G. (2005) Reflective practice and Socratic dialogue. In C. Johns and D. Freshwater (eds), *Transforming Nursing Through Reflective Practice* (2nd edn; pp. 38–54). Oxford, Blackwell Publishing.

White, E. and Winstanley, J. (2010) A randomised controlled trial of clinical supervision: selected findings from a novel Australian attempt to establish the evidence base for causal relationships with quality of care and patient outcomes, as an informed contribution to mental health nursing practice development. *Journal of Research in Nursing*, 15(2), 151–167.

Wilkes, Z. (2006) The student-mentor relationship: a review of the literature. *Nursing Standard*, 20(37), 42–47.

GLOSSARY

5WH Inquiring words such as 'when', 'what', 'why', 'who', 'where' or 'how'.

active listening A form of communication that aids the nurse in listening attentively to the patient and shows the patient they are being listened to.

adapted child The controlled child ego state in transactional analysis.

ambivalence to change Behaviour-change terminology describing mixed motivations to change behaviour.

authenticity To act with genuineness.

authoritarian leadership Leadership style which directs others with little consultation with team members.

authoritative Holding a position of superiority in intervention analysis.

beneficent Having good intent; intending to do good.

boundaries (in nursing) The limits of behaviour which allow a nurse or midwife to have a professional relationship with the person in their care.

catalytic Facilitating problem-solving in intervention analysis.

cathartic Producing a release of tension in intervention analysis.

circular questioning Questions which assist in looking at the issue from a different viewpoint.

classical conditioning Behavioural explanation of the learning of physical reactions to external stimuli.

client-centred therapy Form of therapeutic relating, developed by Carl Rogers, in which the client is empowered to explore and resolve their own needs.

clinical supervision Giving and receiving supervision of practice as a form of reflection.

closing down Method for controlling and reducing high expressed emotion and excitability.

cognitive behavioural therapy (CBT) A therapeutic approach focusing on how a person perceives, interprets and reacts to situations.

conditioning (study of)   Behavioural understanding of learning.

conformity   Adapting one's behaviour, attitude or belief in line with a group identity.

confronting   A position of being challenging in intervention analysis.

critical parent   The controlling and criticising parent ego state in transactional analysis.

degenerate   A destructive communication style in intervention analysis.

democratic leadership   Leadership style which facilitates the involvement of others but retains a decision-making role.

descriptor (educational)   A word in an assignment that indicates what the student is expected to do.

diagnostic overshadowing   Attributing a physical symptom to a learning disability and/or mental health problem.

discrepancy   Between behaviour and values. Outcome sought by motivational interviewers to reveal irrational thinking of person in a state of ambivalence to change.

dyad   A protected pattern of communication involving two people within a group.

dysfunctional thinking   Thinking styles which are unhelpful and lead to maladaptive behaviour.

dysphasia   Difficulty in speaking.

ego state (parent, adult, child)   The attitude of mind a person adopts when communicating with others.

empathy   The ability to enter the perceptual world of the other person.

empowerment   Strategy or philosophy in which the therapeutic goal is to facilitate another's self-care and self-determination.

facilitative   Holding an enabling position in intervention analysis.

game/game-playing   Having an ulterior motive to control others in transactional analysis.

genuineness   Being yourself with your patient.

Heron's six-category intervention analysis   A model for professional interpersonal development, delineating six different styles of interaction.

horizontal organisation   Teamwork consisting of equality of roles: a decentralised power structure.

humanistic Recognising human individualism and freedom to choose.

intersectionality The theory that power structures based on categories such as gender, race, sexuality and class interact and create inequalities, discrimination and oppression.

laissez-faire leadership Leadership style which permits free access to decision-making by team members.

Maslow's hierarchy of needs A humanistic model of personal dependence.

mutuality The degree of shared relating between a nurse and patient.

natural child The carefree ego state in transactional analysis.

negative stroke A negative attention-giving interaction in transactional analysis.

non-directive An approach to counselling which assumes a relationship of equals.

non-maleficent Having no bad intent; intending no harm.

non-verbal attending Reading body language and vocalisations while listening to another.

nurturing parent The caring parent ego state in transactional analysis.

open questioning Questioning style designed to elicit complex answers.

operant conditioning Behavioural explanation for learned behaviour.

paraphrasing Repeating back to a person in your own words what they have just said, to show that you understand their meaning.

paternalistic (medical model) Adopting a position of authoritative protection in relation to patients.

position The attitudinal status adopted by one person in relation to another in an interaction.

positive stroke A positive attention-giving interaction in transactional analysis.

prescriptive Giving instruction in intervention analysis.

prodromal Relating to the period of pathology which precedes symptom appearance.

proxemics 'Personal space', or the proximity of people to each other and the body zones that are acceptable for touching or viewing.

reflective practice Applying reflection on past events to problem-solving in present practice.

reinforcement Presentation of stimuli that strengthen reward-oriented behaviour (positive reinforcement) or avoidance behaviour (negative reinforcement).

revalidation The process of confirming one's continuing professional development with the NMC in order to update one's registration status.

rolling with resistance Therapeutic technique used in motivational interviewing which enables the therapist to avoid confrontation.

scapegoat A person unfairly blamed for the problems of a group.

self-awareness Being conscious of one's own character.

self-care (in nursing) A patient's ability to provide for their own needs.

self-disclosure The technique of sharing experiences to improve mutuality.

self-efficacy The belief that one can control one's own environment; a sense of autonomy.

self-statement An outcome elicited in motivational interviewing and brief intervention in which the interviewee verbalises a key problem.

sequential questioning Questioning style that is often direct and which follows a sequence of events.

six-category intervention analysis, Heron's *See* Heron's six-category intervention analysis

social identity One's identity as defined by group membership.

socialisation The process of developing behaviour, attitudes and beliefs to adapt to one's social environment.

Socratic questioning Pursuing a line of questioning until all the details are revealed.

stroke (positive and negative) Episode of attention-giving in transactional analysis.

supportive An encouraging interaction style in intervention analysis.

sympathy Being affected by the same feeling as another.

transaction An interaction between two people in transactional analysis.

transactional analysis (TA) A model of communication marking the 'positions' of the interactors.

transference A psychoanalytical term meaning the transfer of an emotional relationship from one significant person to another (usually a therapist or carer).

triad A protected communication pattern involving a small group within a group (often a sub-group).

triangulation Common dynamic in which a person acts as peace-maker for two others who have a dispute.

ulterior transaction One position or ego state presenting as another ego state.

unconditional positive regard A humanistic approach in which one adopts a non-judgemental and encouraging attitude in the therapeutic space.

universality A sense of sharing experiences with others.

vicarious learning Learning through watching others.

vocal attending The vocal noises and responses we make during speech and the way we use our voice.

voice prosody Altering voice tonality.

INDEX